Christ Defeats Cancer

Christ Defeats Cancer

by

Scotty McCoy

with editing by

Steve Seitzinger

with a foreword written by

Dr. Steven Toms

Published by CreateSpace

ISBN-13: 978-1542304986
ISBN-10: 1542304989

THIS BOOK IS TO HONOR AND CELEBRATE THE LIFE OF MY DAD, SCOTT G. MCCOY, WHO BATTLED AGAINST A RARE AND AGGRESSIVE FORM OF BRAIN CANCER. THANKFULLY HE HAS BEEN HEALED. THE POWER OF PRAYER IS AMAZING. THANK YOU TO JESUS CHRIST, MY LORD AND SAVIOR. YOU HAVE OBLITEREATED MY DAD'S FORMER CANCER. I LOVE YOU DAD.

ACKNOWLEDGEMENTS

The Family: Thanks to both the McCoy and Seitzinger families for going through this long, exhausting, and emotional journey with us. We got through this together as a family and I know it wasn't easy, but by God's grace and strength we did it!

Our Friends: I want to thank our family friends for being there for us throughout our time of need. Even though things are looking up and everyt hing is going the way God has planned, our friends continue to be a great source of support. They helped us tremendously when we needed them the most. We thank you from the bottom of our hearts.

Jesus Christ: And I saved the best for last. Thanks to our Lord and Savior, Jesus Christ. Because of Him, my dad survived the toughest fight of his life. Jesus provided the miracle for my dad to beat cancer. As the Bible states: "Through Jesus stripes, my dad is healed."

ABOUT THE AUTHOR

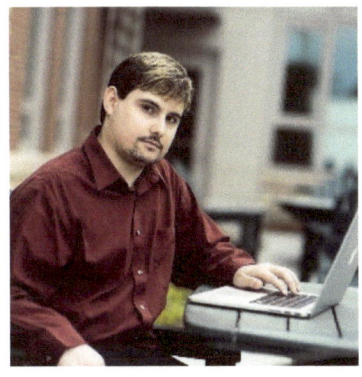 I, Scotty McCoy, was born on December 6, 1989. I am a published author, who has accomplished a lot in my young adult life.

I obtained an Associate's of Applied Science Degree from Luzerne County Community College in Web/Software Development and a Bachelor's of Science Degree from Champlain College in Web/Software Development, as well as a specialized certification in Computer Science from the South Campus of Schuylkill Technology Centers. Despite my educational accomplishments, I am not shy in learning, educating, and challenging myself in new subjects, ventures, and endeavors.

I graduated in 2008 from North Schuylkill High School. I had a teacher named Mrs. Joann Hoppel for English class in 9th and 12th grades. I stated in various interviews, that because of the knowledge obtained in her classes; I retrieved the skills and confidence needed to become a successful author.

I have published two books: *The Ultimate Friday the 13th Trivia Book* and *The Ultimate Halloween Trivia Book*. This is my third book; a biographical novel on my dad's amazing and miraculous defeat of cancer, which has changed my family's lives forever: *Christ Defeats Cancer*.

I appeared on various radio shows, podcasts, television and web series, and in magazines and on

Websites as a celebrity guest to promote my career in writing, such as on the *Return to Camp Blood Radio Show*, *Python's Paradise*, *Klimczak's Killer Collection*, the *Horror Fuel* Website, and in the December 2016 edition of *Popcorn Horror* magazine.

My writing is about the horror genre, where I write about various horror-related topics and subjects. I had two book signings: one in Frackville, Pennsylvania and the other at the King of Prussia Mall.

I had various jobs, including a Software Database Engineer position at Computer Software Incorporated, a Senior PHP Web Application Developer position at GINtech Systems, a supervisory role at Kmart, a cashier position at McDonald's, and a Web Development and Computer Information Systems Tutor, as well as a Peer Mentoring position at Luzerne County Community College. I even start in January 2018 as an online college professor at my alma mater, Champlain College, in the Web/Software Development curriculum where I'll be teaching both programming and theory-related courses.

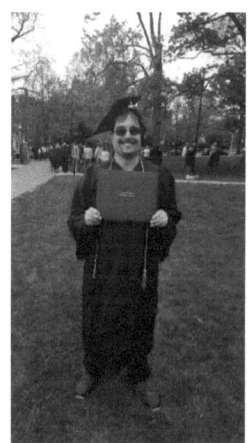

I graduated from Champlain College with a 3.88 GPA as a Summa Cum Laude (Latin Honors) graduate. I had the honor of being inducted into the Alpha Sigma Lambda National Honor Society; the most prestigious honor society for adult students.

I've endured a difficult childhood because of bullying, due to a diagnosis of Tourette's Syndrome. I've demonstrated to people faced with adversity that all things are possible through Christ. So, if you want to do something, just work hard, focus, and put your mind to it and your dreams can come true.

Sincerely,

Scotty McCoy

Scotty McCoy
Author, *Christ Defeats Cancer*

ABOUT SCOTT G. MCCOY

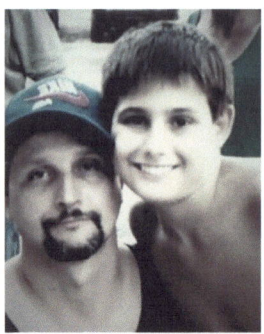

Scott McCoy was always quiet when growing up, but he was caring and would do anything for anybody. Scott enjoyed playing sports, especially baseball, and was an amazing pitcher. He always ate healthily and made a habit of using his brother Ken's weights to work out. His favorite meal was spaghetti as a kid and it still is. My mom even remembers when my grandmother told her that my dad would grow up to be a minister as he loved going to Sunday School and church.

My dad was always a hardworking man who would do the simplest of things for anybody in need, such as unfreezing his mom's pipes during the winter months. He was the type of worker that didn't mind "getting his hands dirty" by doing manual labor work. He worked for 28 years at the Frackville, Pennsylvania state prison. He also did catering on the side, and has catered countless spaghetti and meatloaf dinners for Zion's Reformed United Church of Christ.

After speaking with my dad's sister, Marci; she told me a story that describes my dad's growing up years. My aunt Marci is his older sister, and she reports always tormenting and picking on him. At one point, their mom, my grandmother, told my dad, "don't ever hit girls." Marci used this to her advantage, until one day my dad said, enough was enough and he hit her back in self-defense. Marci, shocked, ran to her parents (my grandparents), and told them my dad hit her back. As Marci told me this story, I could hear my grandmother's voice as she laughed "Ah ha, ah ha, now you did it! I told you to stop picking on him, so you had it coming for not listening!" As Marci concluded the story, she told me her parents were right. She had it coming!

My dad was always concerned about other people. It was easier for him to put others before himself. He did this ever since he was a kid. His dad always told him that big boys should not cry. So, he would hold back his tears during sad moments that would happen in his life. After speaking about this topic with my aunt Marci, she encouraged him that it was okay to cry, because "real men cry." I remember when my grandfather passed away, my dad wouldn't cry, but you can tell he wanted too. The same response came when his mother and brothers, Ken and Joe, passed away.

My dad went through a lot of heartache later in his life, such as losing both of his parents and two brothers. He walks in peace; knowing they all are in Heaven with our Lord and Savior, Jesus Christ. When they all passed away, he never once cried in front of people. But, I believe he fought back tears, because it was his way of trying to show everybody he was strong.

I remember when my grandfather, who was in the hospital, passed away. While in the hospital he made me promise that when he died, I wouldn't cry. Well, he passed away and at his funeral, I bawled my eyes out. My dad saw how upset I was, so he tried to make me smile by telling a joke. My dad stated, "Didn't you promise pap you wouldn't cry when he passed away?" I responded with a whimper in my voice, "Yeah!" My dad followed up by saying "Well, you just broke that promise!" The funny thing is that his reminder put a smirk on my face and I didn't cry for the remainder of the funeral. I knew my pap wanted me to be happy and to be comforted by the fact that he was at peace and no longer suffering.

Marci told me another story about my dad, pertaining me. This shows how my dad's desire and humility in wanting me to become a man. In 1991, I was two years old. During that time, the laws weren't as strict as they are today. My dad brought me to my grandmother's house. My grandmother said to Marci, when telling the story, that my dad brought me to her house on a cool day without wearing a coat. She asked my dad, "Where is his coat?" He replied, "My son is not going to grow up to become a wimp!"

He always showed determination and we knew this was God's strength, allowing my dad to survive emergency brain surgery and a major stroke, complete radiation therapy and rehabilitation, and defeat brain cancer. The persevering mindset my dad grew up with and developed was helpful in his battle.

I had an amazing childhood and father. My father amazes me to this day. He is so strong and brave, which I believe were essential in helping him to survive brain cancer. Our Christian beliefs were instrumental in his victory and recovery as well. My dad is such an inspiration to me and my family, and hopefully to everyone who reads his success story.

His battle with cancer, which I posted on Facebook went viral; and I hope this inspired people to believe, have faith, and stay positive. With this type of inspiration, my dad believes that other people battling cancer will discover hope and the will to fight until they achieve victory.

I don't think I could go through everything he did this past year and survive. I would be too scared to face the battle. I know if it weren't for God; even watching my dad would have been impossible. But thanks to God, I could watch my dad not just fight for his life, but also survive and eventually thrive.

My dad is not any ordinary person. He is a strong Christian, who permitted Jesus to overcome Satan's curse that was placed upon him and our family. Dad told my aunt Marci "I will survive this fight. I am not ready to leave my wife and son." Once again, he was thinking of others and not of himself. My dad continued, "I'm not afraid to die, I just don't want to leave my family." Family is important to my dad. He would do everything possible to maintain it.

All my dad wanted was for his friends and family to be by his side, and boy did he have that. The medical staff joked about having a celebrity in the hospital, because of the huge support system he had. I jokingly said to the staff, "You do have a celebrity here! I'm a famous published author!" My dad then laughed and jokingly said "This is The Scotty McCoy Hour" which he often said, when I talked about myself because of my ego. HA!

Two days after the surgery, my dad had the stroke. He was in the Intensive Care Unit (ICU). Even though his life was hanging by a thread, he was still thinking of others before himself. He asked Marci if she could order Centiole's, a famous local pizza place known for their homemade pizza pies, to serve the nurses. He also asked Marci to order my mom flowers.

During his recovery, his determination was to get well. He had amazing nurses, including Julie and Heather, both of whom he talks about to this day. He cannot thank them enough for how well they did their job to nurse him back to health. He surprised and amazed the entire medical team at Geisinger Medical Center in Danville, Pennsylvania about how fast he was recovering and getting back on his feet.

Various family members and even friends told him, "Scott, you have helped so many people in your life. It is now time for us to be able to give back to you." Even though my dad didn't like hearing those words, and often resisted us when we would do something for him that he wanted to do, he appreciated the love and support from his family and friends. He eventually got used to it. Although he had no choice in the matter. HA!

A year has gone by, and I, as his son, still cry myself to sleep some nights after thinking of the suffering that my dad went through and how his life has changed. This made me realize that life is too short and never to take it for granted. Don't just tell your loved ones that you love them, but show them because you never know when they'll take their last breath or something tragic, sudden, and unexpected can happen and change your life.

At the time of diagnosis, my dad was only 54 years old. Too young to have something like this happen to him, so you never know when something can happen. Just realize that in a blink of an eye, your life can change forever. You are never too young to die or to get a life-threatening condition. Thankfully, my dad is still alive and I will never take him for granted like I used to.

To this day, I look at my dad and want to cry, even as I am writing this. I realize in the moment, I almost lost my father. But as the fighter that he is and through the perseverance and power given to him by our Lord Jesus Christ, Glioblastoma has been defeated.

One thing cancer has learned this past year is that when you come face to face with Christ, you stand no chance of winning. As Scott McCoy's spirit has been filled with the undying love and purity of our Lord Jesus and His divine healing; Satan has been defeated once again. Amen!

FOREWORD

Glioblastoma multiforme (GBM) is the most devastating cancer of the central nervous system in adults. The disease seems to arise from the structural supporting cells of the brain through the accumulation of genetic defects (mutations) likely caused by genetic material being altered by environmental exposures such as certain viruses we all contract in our lifetimes.

These genetic mistakes in a single cell divide and grow, until a mass of billions of cancer cells invade the eloquent structure of the brain like a weed. In short, nothing we do in our daily lives seems to cause (or prevent) someone from the misfortune of developing a GBM.

In the United States alone, 12,000 new cases of GBM are diagnosed each year. Currently, standard treatment consists of maximal safe surgical resection or a diagnostic biopsy, followed by radiotherapy with concomitant daily temozolomide chemotherapy. Despite these efforts, most patients die within 1 to 2 years of diagnosis.

It was with this background (and my own family's history of cancer) that I began my journey as a brain surgeon and cancer researcher 30 years ago. After years of arduous training, often sacrificing time from family for patients or the laboratory, we have begun to make progress on this dreaded disease on several fronts, from vaccines and other modulators of the immune system, to electrical fields that stop cancer cell division. Some of these advances have led to the doubling of survival over the past 20 years and are leading to our first long term survivors for this disease.

I had the good fortune to meet and take care of Mr. McCoy as he began his own personal cancer journey in September of 2016. He has done very well since his surgery and will hopefully continue to do well in the months and years to come. His story and success inspired me to continue the long hours in the operating room and the laboratory, hoping that we can continue to understand the complexities of these rogue brain cells that develop into the weed we call GBM so that one day I will not need to give bad haircuts to try to extract these invaders from the delicate structures of the human brain.

Steven A. Toms, MD

INTRODUCTION

Faith. Strength. Perseverance. Determination. Love. Survivor. What do these six words have in common? Life! And a second question as it pertains to this book; is who do these six words represent? Scott George McCoy. He is the prime example of what faith, strength, perseverance, determination, love, and survivor stands for in the heart of a person, who surrenders their life to the Lord Jesus Christ. And this is his biography, a tribute of sorts, to Scott, in the hope of showing the world what a fighter truly looks like, but more importantly, what a miracle looks like.

This biography will be told from the viewpoint of Scott's son, Scotty McCoy, the author of this book, and what he, his mom, Lisa, and his entire family went through after Scott was diagnosed with a rare, aggressive form of brain cancer, known as Glioblastoma. This type of cancer is classified as incurable, yet somewhat treatable. This book unfolds the bumpy, sometimes uncertain, yet satisfying road to recovery.

Even though Scott is a fighter and a miracle, he couldn't have fought and been given the will to fight and defeat cancer if it wasn't for our Lord and Savior, Jesus Christ. Thanks to the strength imparted to Scott, by his faith in the Lord and the support of his loving family, Scott has defeated cancer. But more importantly, Christ gave him the fight and willpower to even try.

Reading this introduction, we all know the outcome, especially for those who have followed the story on Facebook. However, what many may not know is the mental, emotional, and physical toll it took, not just on Scott, but his entire family, close friends, and strangers that follow Scotty as an author from all corners of the world. Much gratitude to those in the family of God, who don't even really know him, but prayed for him as a fellow brother in Christ.

This novel, starting with chapter one, will give the reader a glimpse of life before cancer, leading up to the diagnosis, and then ending with his miraculous defeat of cancer. Few know how powerful prayer is, but if it wasn't for the numerous, consistent, and fervent prayers offered on behalf of my dad, and the amazing, supernatural, and unconditional love of our Lord and Savior, my dad would not be here today and this book would have a different title. But thankfully, this book is to honor, celebrate, and embrace the life of Scott G. McCoy, and to glorify the Lord Jesus Christ, without whom, my dad would not have continued life on this earth.

You'll see in depth details and graphical analyses on everything that transpired from the time the symptoms slowly, but surely began to show till the present day. Details that I have witnessed personally, as well as information obtained from family and friends will also be told. The story you are about to read is something that will not only shock you, but amaze you. The miracles my dad experienced and the signs our family witnessed by the Lord Jesus Christ will be revealed. We pray this encourages you to remember there is always hope, even if the future looks bleak.

In the end, you will be taken on a journey; a journey not only of survival, but "thrival." "Thrival" is a word we made up to describe joyous victory. Dr. Steven Toms, the neurosurgeon who took care of my father, stated out of his own mouth that Scott G. McCoy is nothing less than a miracle and nothing more than a survivor. Prepare yourself to be exposed to the power of prayer, the unconditional love of our Lord, the bravery and courage of my dad, and most importantly, the reality of how *Christ Defeats Cancer*.

TABLE OF CONTENTS

CHAPTER 1: ONE MONTH PRIOR

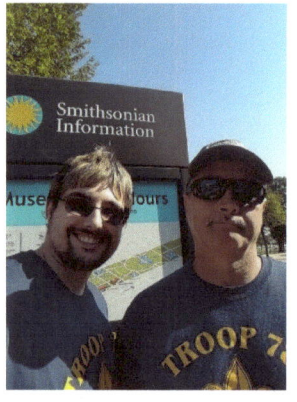 The date was August 6, 2016 and we had a Seitzinger family reunion at my mom's cousins, Lori and Tom's, campground. It was a fun event; however, it was too hot outside and I started to feel ill.

The next day after the reunion, I was going with my dad to meet a former WWE superstar, Damien Sandow, in Allentown, Pennsylvania, but had to cancel, because it was so hot outside at the reunion the previous day. Due to the excessive heat and the sun gleaming on me, I woke up in the morning with a major headache. I remember with the sun gleaming on my head, I felt like I was getting overheated and needed some shade, but it was so hot outside that I was unable to shield myself from the heat.

Because of the extensive heat, I was kind of complaining about wanting to go home. The reunion was outside, of course, and was an all-day event. Even with complaining about wanting to go home, my dad told me that we can't and we stayed at the campground until nighttime.

I remember vividly that my dad and I had a big argument at the reunion. We never made up and I never apologized for that argument or my behavior. But it is something I still regret to this day, because little did I know, the tumor that was inside of my dad's head was already growing. I never expected my dad to get a tumor, especially a rare, aggressive, and fast-growing one that would be cancerous. I always thought of my dad as being immortal. Even though no one is, I guess I thought this because he was my father. Who would have thought that something like this would happen to him?

We went home that night and the next morning we were fine. All was well. There were no arguments or strife, because we have had plenty of previous arguments and tiffs. This was bound to happen. We were too much alike. My mom always called us twins when I was younger because we always argued. Nothing major nor physical, just your typical father-son disagreements. I never got spanked as a kid, however, I did lose the privilege of watching the next episode of WWE Monday Night Raw on television. Yes, I lost wrestling when I got punished as a child. I lost wrestling, because it was something I loved. It worked and I certainly behaved more frequently.

Growing up, I had amazing parents. The funny thing is my dad was always the big softie, where my mom was always the strict one. If I wanted something, anything at all, my dad would get it for me. I just needed to say in a sweet voice with my handsome smile "Please, daddy" and I got it. Even when I went off to college in 2008 and my dad took me food shopping for my apartment, I'd say "Please, daddy" and he'd say "Alright, put it in the cart. But no more! We're going to the check out!" Let's just say I got more. HA! I never took advantage of my dad. I really love him. He is just an amazing father and would do anything for me, because it is how he showed his affection. I wouldn't say I never got disciplined, because I did. I got discipled, because it was also my dad's way of showing me how much he cared.

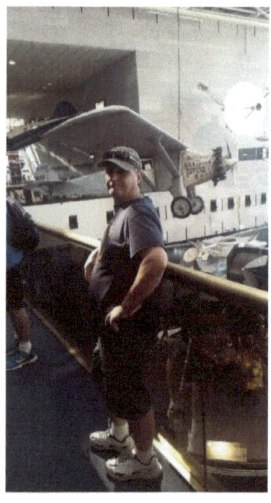

Approximately a week or so before the symptoms began on August 20, 2016, my dad and I went with the Boy Scouts on a bus trip to Washington DC. Everything was going great and we got some amazing pictures together too. Plus, my dad got to see the exhibit of The Spirit of St. Louis at the Smithsonian Institute's National Air and Space Museum. The Spirit of St. Louis was a custom-built, single-engine, and single-seated monoplane that was flown by Charles Lindbergh from May 20, 1927 to May 21, 1927 on the first solo non-stop transatlantic flight from Long Island, New York to Paris, France. He even got to get his picture taken by it and I was so glad to have spent that moment with my dad to see the exhibit with him. This is a moment I'll truly cherish and remember for the rest of my life.

Roughly about a week or so before the diagnosis, my dad wasn't acting quite himself. We thought he was just being goofy at first, and then it started to become worrisome. He just didn't seem to be his usual, caring self anymore. We weren't really alarmed to the point of taking to a hospital or anything. For example, it started out with minor things, that were funny and even cute at first. For instance, he would go outside to cut the grass and find out he didn't have any shoes on or he would go to drive to the store or to a Boy Scout meeting and he wouldn't have his pants on; only his boxers. We just thought my dad was being a little goofy. But we never imagined that he was beginning to manifest a neurological or psychological deficit. We certainly never entertained the fact that he had a brain tumor.

At the end of August 2016, we were in Wal Mart over in Shamokin, Pennsylvania, and just doing some casual shopping. This was the first moment I can vividly remember something being wrong with my dad's personality, but it wasn't until our drive home. However, while inside Wal Mart he dropped a can of zesty pickles when he tried to put it in the cart. He came over to me and started laughing and said, "They'll soon be paging for clean up in the pickle aisle." I asked him why and he responded by saying "I dropped a pickle jar and it got all over the floor." He didn't even tell anyone, but just left quickly and continued laughing. Again, this was not my true dad's personality, but I just thought of it as a humorous situation, not a neurological disaster. The thing is, he dropped the pickle jar while picking it up, because the tumor was pressing on various parts of his brain that helped him move his extremities (hands, arms, legs, and feet). We just didn't know at the time the reason he really dropped the pickle jar in Wal Mart. People suffering from a tumor inside of their brain will act in ways contrary to their true selves. You won't think normally and will start slowly, but surely losing mobility functions.

Then, on the drive home from Wal Mart, my dad would just become a danger to himself and to others as well. My dad was driving, my mom was in the passenger seat, and I was in the back. My dad was literally all over the road, crossing the center yellow line, going to the opposite side of the road, etc. Let's just say my mom and I were quite nervous and were beginning to think something was up with dad, but we still weren't smart enough to understand or even comprehend that something mentally and/or neurologically was wrong with him. My dad then drove right through a red light. It is unlike my dad to be so dangerous. It wasn't even a yellow light. I might have been ok with that, but it was solid red and had been that way for at least a minute or two. My dad went through it and me and my mom told him about it. He just shrugged it off and joked. I told him "Do you think the cops will pull us over?" He responded, "We'll find out in a minute if we see flashing lights!" That's not a way my dad would ever respond to a situation like that. He didn't even show concern that he could've killed us or somebody ese. I told my dad "Can you please pull over and let me drive the rest of the way home?" He refused to let me, so my mom chimed in saying "If you can't see the road, then just put on your headlights." He responded, "What makes you think that I can't see the road?" Thankfully, we got home safe and sound that night, although it was quite alarming and concerning for us to say the least.

My dad worked the spring, summer, and fall months, usually between March or April until October. He would do landscaping work with his friends, whom he retired with, John and Dan. Dan would drive to our house and my dad would drive them both to the area they had to go to for the job that day and meet up with John. Dan would tell us after my dad's initial diagnosis that he was afraid of being in the car with my dad. My dad even stated to me after everything was said and done, "I was actually starting to be scared to drive. I never will drive if I feel like I am a danger to myself or others. I didn't realize how bad it was till after the tumor was removed." He didn't realize his driving capability was compromised, at least not until everything was all said and done. That's what a brain tumor tends to do to a person. It makes you feel normal, but you really aren't acting as normal as you think you are. We noticed things here and there, but again, nothing serious enough to cause us concern that something was medically wrong. It just goes to show, a brain tumor is just so subtle sometimes, in terms of how some individuals feel physically, emotionally, and mentally.

      As the days went on, my dad became increasingly different as a person. He basically wasn't himself at all anymore. It got more noticeable, but to me and my mom, we still thought nothing bad would happen to him. After all, he's Scott McCoy. He's strong, young, and healthy. Nothing would happen to him, but then come September, we got a phone call; a phone call from my dad's close friend who worked with him as a landscaper. This phone call from his retired friend might have just saved my dad's life.

CHAPTER 2: THE MONTH OF

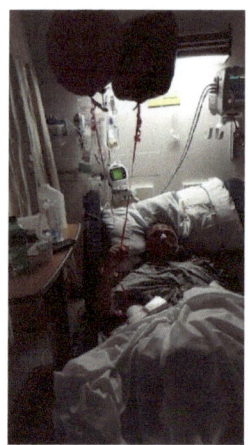

On September 13, 2016, we took my dad to the emergency room. My dad wasn't much of a hospital guy, so I threatened to call an ambulance and even had 911 dialed on my phone. This ultimately got him to agree to go. Why? Because we got a phone call from his good friend that he worked with as a landscaper. John's call might be the reason my dad is still alive, because John brought it to our attention. It was as if God had given us this gift as a warning, so my dad could get and seek the medical attention that he needed.

My mom was down the road at my aunt Lou Ann's house visiting. My dad, on the other hand, was working with John landscaping. My dad would work in the scorching heat for 12 hours a day and roughly five days a week. He loved every minute of it as well. My mom even realized my dad was always tired, but she only thought it was due to his excessive work schedule.

While visiting my aunt Lou Ann, my mom received a phone call from John, describing my dad's odd behavior while landscaping. "He wasn't his normal self," said John. My dad was already home from work, but he drove down to the church where he had his Boy Scouts meetings, since he is the Scoutmaster. My mom barged into the door and asked where my dad was. I am all nervous, not knowing if he was in a car crash, and yelling at my mom to tell me what was going on. She eventually told me that John called and told me what he said and that we needed to rush my dad to the emergency room. I was scared, but hopeful that it wasn't anything too serious. I just thought it was possibly Lyme's disease, since he worked outdoors. Or maybe even a mini stroke as a worst-case scenario.

So, we got my dad to the hospital and they did some tests on him. They settled with dehydration, as he was dehydrated. They gave him fluids, until he got his strength back. While my dad worked with John and Dan, he would take water with him. However, he didn't drink enough, so therefore the doctors settled on him being dehydrated. They ended up releasing him, but my uncle Steve wasn't satisfied with that diagnosis as he knew something neurologically was wrong. For those who do not know my uncle Steve, he is extremely knowledgeable about medical issues He currently works as a Christian counselor. He used to be a physician assistant as well. But at the time, Steve let it go, and even though he was unsatisfied with the diagnosis, he permitted my dad to come back home.

On September 14, 2016, my uncle Steve came up with his wife, my aunt Jeanette. He did some neurological tests on my dad and based on his testing, something was wrong inside his brain. To make sure that he was understanding the tests he found online, he performed the tests on my mom, as well as on myself. My mom and I both passed the tests which showed that our brains were functioning appropriately. However, my dad failed his neurological tests, which had Steve 100 percent certain that my dad wasn't just "dehydrated" as the doctors stated the previous night.

We rushed my dad back to the Shamokin hospital, telling them that it was unacceptable to release my dad on a dehydration diagnosis without following up with a CT Scan. They performed a CT Scan and BAM! The results were in! They said he had a brain tumor that was most likely cancerous. They said it was a large tumor and they were going to rush him to Geisinger in Danville, where he'll need to be given an MRI to get a better understanding of what the tumor exactly was. They were then going to perform emergency surgery first thing in the morning.

Steve drove me to Geisinger, while my mom rode in the ambulance with my dad. After hearing the doctor stating my dad had a brain tumor, I screamed. I screamed so loud, as I began to tremble with fear. My mom was silenced. No words to say. No emotions to feel. She was just in complete and utter shock. Steve tried calming me down. He held me in his arms and reminded me, "They said it is operable, not inoperable, which means that he can still beat this." As he told me this, all I could think about was my dad's tumor and how I have been horribly treating my father lately. I knew it might be too late to make it up to him and begin treating him right. I did apologize for the way I had been treating him lately. I gave him a kiss on the forehead, and then drove with Steve to the main unit of Geisinger Medical Center in Danville, Pennsylvania. It's amazing how something bad like this makes you realize how short life is and that, in a blink of an eye, your entire vision of life changes. So, tell everyone you love and that is close to you that you love them, give them a hug and a kiss, because in a split second, your life can change and you can either lose them or be on the verge of saying your final goodbyes.

My dad was being transported from the Shamokin hospital to the main unit of Geisinger in Danville via an ambulance, while my mom rode in the back with him. While I was in the car with my uncle Steve, I was crying. I was bawling my eyes out, barely audible as the tears ran down my cheeks. My whole body was shaking. My hands were trembling in fear, and my heart palpitating to a beat of its own drum. I swear I thought I was going to have an anxiety attack. I was on the brink of hyperventilating; that's how badly my body was shaking. Steve led me in prayer. Even though I was unable to speak properly due to the outburst of sadness coming vocally from my mouth, the Lord knew what I was trying to say and would use that to answer my first of many prayers in the forthcoming months. This is the point in time that I needed to put my dad's life and my trust and faith in the Lord. No ifs, ands, or buts about it, my faith is about to be tested like it never has been before.

My dad was calmer about this entire ordeal, more than my mom and me. We didn't know what to say or think. My dad ended up telling us "Relax, guys. It's not a death sentence!" A few months after, he would tell us "It may not be a death sentence, but it is a life sentence!"

Upon arrival to the hospital, we located my dad's room where my mom was by his side. They took my dad back to the room where they'd give him his MRI to see what type of brain tumor we're dealing with and to confirm if it was a cancerous tumor. Once we reunited with my mom, Steve left for the night and my mom and I spent the next several weeks, 24 hours a day and seven days a week, in the hospital sleeping in the waiting room. My mom and I barely slept or ate. I cannot speak exactly for her, but I hadn't eaten a thing or slept a wink in a little over a week. Other family members and friends would also spend the night in the waiting room with my mom and I throughout the forthcoming weeks on random, rotating nights, which by the way was kind of fun, despite the horrible situation, which I'll get into in a little bit.

I recently told my parents what I said to my dad, both unaware of what I said. My mom wasn't in the room and my dad was fast asleep. My dad doesn't remember what I said as he was medicated to keep him comfortable, relaxed, and rested, but after I told him we cast out the curse I put upon myself. However, I only did it because I felt like my dad doesn't deserve what he was going through. I told my dad "Dad, I don't know if you can hear me, because of the amounts of medicine that you are currently on. But you don't deserve what you are going through. I wish I had this tumor that you have. I wish I was the one in this hospital where you are right now. I wish I could trade places with you because you have done more for me than I could for you in my entire lifetime, and this would just be a small price I'd pay for you." You know when you love someone like I do my dad when you want to take his spot in the hospital and suffer like he was. He was suffering and about to undergo major brain surgery, and I felt powerless to do anything to help him.

After this when my dad was awake, I spoke to him regarding a major life decision that I had been thinking about. I was contemplating dropping out of college, due to the overwhelming situation my dad and family were going through. I talked to him about this, and not thinking of himself, he said to me "When I get better, I want to be at your commencement ceremony in Vermont. I cannot go if you drop out so you pass those classes. If you don't quit and pass those classes, that will be the best medicine for me and give me the motivation to get better by May 2017."

The doctor and neurosurgeon, Dr. Steven Toms, came in around six in the morning, with me and my mom sitting by my dad's bedside all night long. I couldn't sleep, nor could my mom. Once Dr. Toms came in he described to us what exactly this tumor was. It was called Glioblastoma and it is a rare, aggressive form of brain cancer. He went into details of what exactly the tumor was and what'll happen in the coming months and years.

After the in-depth analysis on what Glioblastoma was and the road my dad would have to take to get better, Dr. Toms then told us exactly what we're dealing with in terms of my dad's tumor size and his opinions on the tumor. He told us this tumor was the size of a man's fist, which if you are a male and make a fist, the entire size of said fist is the mass inside my dad's skull. Dr. Toms said that this tumor was the largest he had seen in his entire career as a neurosurgeon, which at the time was a tad longer than 29 years. He continued to tell us that if left undiagnosed and unnoticed, my dad would have fallen asleep one night and he wouldn't have woken up. He told us my dad literally had less than a month left to live if this tumor was left undiagnosed. He even told us this tumor is that aggressive that it literally grew to this size since August, which means all the signs we and others have noticed were the signs of the tumor growing. Yes, this tumor grew that large in only a month's time, which is unheard of. It's hard to believe something so evil and deadly was living in my dad's brain. Satan cast this tumor onto my dad, and he may have won the battle in terms of giving this to my dad, but he was going to lose the war, because of who lives inside of my dad: Jesus. My dad, let's just say, put Satan in his place due to his undying love and faith in our Lord and Savior, Jesus Christ.

Anyways, I was shocked at the revelation of what we were dealing with. Not knowing for a month that this tumor grew from nothing into something so massive. It was something I never expected to hear about my dad. I mean he's my father and he is my hero. I always had this funny thought that my dad'll never die and nothing bad would ever happen to him because, well, he's my father.

However, the news that Dr. Toms told us next had both my mom and I relieved and gave us a sly of hope and the sign we needed from God, so we could get through this, especially after the devastating news that we have been receiving the past 12 hours.

He said he is confident that he can remove between 95 to 99 percent of the tumor, since it is in a spot that isn't around any inoperable parts of the brain. After the brain surgery is completed and he heals up, he'll then begin radiation and chemotherapy treatments. He gave us the rundown of what'll happen leading up to and after surgery. I then began calling my entire family that morning and letting them know that my dad is about to undergo major brain surgery. I told them the time he'll begin getting prepped for surgery, and slowly, but surely throughout that morning my entire family, along with amazing family friends came to the hospital and waited with us in the waiting room for hours upon hours until surgery was completed.

While prepping for surgery, the nurse made a comment to my dad about the calluses on his feet. My dad responded to her in a sarcastic, funny, and yet serious way saying "Lady, that is the least of my problems!" My dad then called over Dr. Toms and asked him if he had a minute. Dr. Toms said "Yes, Scott. What do you need?" My dad then followed up by saying, "I need to ask you two questions before we get started." He continued, "My first question is 'are you a Christian?'" Dr. Toms told him that he was. My dad then continued, "The second question I have is 'do you believe in miracles?'" Dr. Toms replied "Yes!" My dad then said, "Let's make one happen!" Dr. Toms then smiled as if he said that the miracle will take place as my dad requested.

During the time of surgery, there were approximately 20+ chairs to be sat in, with the entire McCoy and Seitzinger clan filling them all up. As we had to wait roughly six hours until surgery was done, we had to find some way to keep us occupied and how did we do that? We laughed together, we cried together, and yes, we even prayed together. In attendance during the duration of the six hours of surgery, awaiting to hear the good news of a successful surgery, was me, my mom, my aunts Lou Ann, Lesley, Jeanette, Marci, and Candi, my uncles Kirk, Ron, Steven, Joe, and Dave, and my cousins Jennifer, David and his wife, Amanda, and Matthew. Also, family friends, Lisa, Kenny, Chrissy, my mom's aunt Darlene, John, Dan, and Pastor Mark were in attendance.

Amazing family friends, Kenny and Lisa, brought everyone donuts from Dunkin' Donuts during the surgery which was an amazing gesture. I didn't eat for three days at that time, and my mom tried getting me to eat a donut. I tried, but I ended up throwing it up as my stomach was in knots and I couldn't keep it down. It's friends like them that helped us get through this. It's the small things that mean the most.

As we were waiting in the lobby, I spoke to my aunt Marci. I asked her "Why is this happening to my dad? Why is God allowing this to happen?" She responded, "Everything happens for a reason, but we'll never know that reason until we take our last breath." As she told me this, I understood that my dad and our family's lives are being tested. Our faith as a family is being tested and it is not just going to be our prayers that would help him through this, but our faith and love in the Lord Jesus Christ that would not just help my dad defeat this horrid disease, but also get us as a family to cope with the situation at hand. I have an amazing family, and together we were determined in helping my dad get through the worst time of his life.

After I spoke with Marci, as my dad is now in surgery, it was time to call upon my dad's healing and pray as a family for my dad in the front lobby. We all held hands in a circle, while my uncle Steve, aunt Jeanette, and Pastor Mark led in prayer. I was screaming so loud I think the entire hospital heard me crying out to the Lord and screaming, as the tears flowed from my eyes and down my cheeks. My aunt Marci had her arms around my neck while I sat in the chair, whispering in my ear "It's going to be alright, Scotty. Stay strong, your dad will be fine." I wanted to believe her, but I was just so skeptical. It wasn't because I wanted my dad to die, it was because the enemy, Satan, was wanting me to believe my dad would succumb during surgery and be discouraged with his condition.

After we prayed, we got an unbelievable sign from God. A man walks out of the bathroom and we cannot see his face. I go to my mom "Is that daddy?" She gave me this look probably thinking "Scotty, why would you even say something like that?" Everyone in the lobby looked and it was an exact, identical doppelganger of my dad. He had the same height, body build, his hands in his jean shorts, which my dad always did, hair color, and most shockingly, the same, exact hat my dad owns. I took that as a sign from God saying, "Your dad will be alright, and he's going to be coming back to you and your family as strong as ever!" The funny thing is, I still have the video of that guy on my phone and continue to show people who know my dad and they agree 100 percent that if they walked by him, they'd have said hi to him thinking he was my dad.

After this incident, we even got a bigger sign. A whole bunch of doppelgangers. We began seeing family members and friends of people we know throughout the hospital. Even someone who looked like my aunt Jeanette, just a little heavier. HA! Jen didn't like that lookalike when we mentioned it! We even saw the exact lookalike of my mom's best friend, Laura's, ex-husband, Carl. Short, thin, and bald. Totally creepy, yet totally funny!

Dr. Toms came out approximately six hours later and asked us if everyone is present. I'm shaking in my chair and realized that my aunts Lou Ann and Lesley are missing. Leave it to them two to be shopping in the gift shop right down the hallway. I run, screaming to them, "Pook, Les, Dr. Toms is here, surgeries over, hurry up!" I never saw Lou Ann run so fast. HA! Upon getting them back to the lobby, Dr. Toms told us the surgery was a success and my dad's condition will improve somedays and may even decline other days as his brain has been through a lot. They removed 95 to 99 percent of the tumor like he said they would and the remaining 1 to 5 percent of the tumor must be removed from the brain with radiation and chemotherapy, which he was confident would completely remove his cancer cells and he'd become cancer free due to the minimal amounts of cancer left in his brain.

Thankfully, the surgery was a complete and utter success. By the grace of God, my dad has undergone successful brain surgery. Something not many people are strong enough to even contemplate doing. Granted, my dad had no choice. He either got the surgery or died from the tumor and knowing my dad, he wasn't letting cancer nor Satan succeed and have victory. My dad, with Jesus on his side, was going to fight and by God, he fought and a majority of the tumor was removed.

Right after the surgery was completed and he was recovering in the recovery room, the nurse asked my dad if he needed anything for the pain. My dad replied "The only one who can take my pain away is my wife. She is in the waiting room; can you please go get her?" My dad told me that he was carrying on so much after surgery to see my mom, his wife that he thought the doctor would let the nurse go and get her. The nurse evidently responded with "I wish my husband would say that about me!"

My dad was being wheeled out from the recovery room post-surgery, as my mom and aunt Marci were there watching him being wheeled through the hallway and back to his room. Marci told me that she will never get out of her mind the look of fear and pain in my dad's eyes. As my dad made eye contact with his sister, he said "It hurt so bad!" Marci grabbed my dad's hand, fighting back tears, and told him "I know it did, but you'll be fine!" He smiled which indicated, "Yes I will be!"

Dr. Toms told us that my dad would need to get an MRI every two to three months after he completes radiation. It is a way to monitor the tumor's regrowth process because if it were to regrow, they'd be able to catch it early and kill it again before it becomes as large as it was this time around. He even told us this type of brain cancer is not curable and can and most likely will come back at some point in his life, but it doesn't mean that it cannot be removed again. However, that is something Dr. Toms is telling us in the natural as a medical practitioner. We, as spiritual, religious Christians know the power of prayer and miracles. We know our Lord's power, so we are not confessing the regrowth of the tumor and are confessing my dad's ultimate healing of brain cancer so the tumor will never regrow again in my dad's entire lifetime.

Even though the surgery had been completed and was a complete and utter success, we all think my dad's in the clear, right? We think that my dad is now on the road to recovery, right?   That he'll begin his radiation and chemotherapy treatments in a few weeks, right? Wrong! We had a setback happen that we hadn't seen coming!

The past few days, our family has been through so much and Satan kept putting us through the ringer. And Satan threw in a curveball with this sick, twisted game he is playing with my dad's life and our entire family's emotions. Well, this hurdle Satan threw our way is just something that we'll fight back against as well. However, this newfound curse that Satan put on my dad would be something that would make the next year even more mentally and emotionally draining.

CHAPTER 3: POST-SURGERY

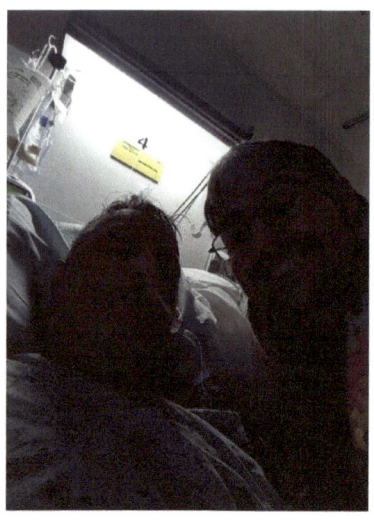

The surgery was a success and my dad was in the recovery room, knocked out from the anesthesia, for the rest of the day.

Everyone got my dad cards and balloons. He even got cards from my friends and fans from other countries, to which he said sarcastically and jokingly, "Who do I know from The Netherlands?"

My cousin Derek always got cards or balloons from my dad for his birthday that wouldn't make sense as a joke, such as "Congratulations on the new house" or "It's a Girl." My cousin Derek got my dad a balloon that said, "It's a Girl" and everyone kept asking who had a baby. One night, my dad woke up in the middle of the night and the balloon was beginning to freak him out. That next morning, the balloon was gone. No one knew where the balloon went and to this day, we never discovered the whereabouts of the balloon.

We could go see him in his room, although they told us he most likely won't be responsive as much. It wasn't anything serious, just from the anesthesia, which they had to use a lot of because of the type of surgery it was. They did need to use just enough so his body can be attested by the surgeons to make sure that he is okay and the surgery goes smoothly. This is done mainly to check his vitals and make sure that, when operating on the brain, nothing major has been touched in the brain. Obviously, nothing major was done to the brain, or so we thought!

On September 16, 2016, one day after the surgery, my dad was waking up and the entire family has surrounded his bedside. My dad kept making his corny jokes that he always does, even one where he was wearing this object with a red light on his finger and he goes "E.T. Go Home," to which my aunt Jeanette thought was hilarious. The doctor came in and he asked him "Who is the president?" At the time, it was Barack Obama, but my dad jokingly stated, as he always does to make a bad situation humorous, "Trump." The doctor laughed and responded, "Not yet!"

My dad told us this story of something that had happened to him during the surgery that put us all in awe. Based on the story my dad told us and what he witnessed, while under the anesthesia, what happened to my dad was something spiritual. Something Holy. Something Godly!

My dad said he felt them drilling into his head, mainly due to the anesthesia not completely knocking him out due to the doctors needing to provide some leverage to his body to see how he interacts throughout the operation. He said he saw gold dust above his head spinning like in a kaleidoscope that gave him peace and comfort. He thought that he was dying and going to Heaven during that moment, but realized he never crossed over into Heaven when he woke up as he doesn't remember seeing Jesus, angels, friends or family, or even anything directly related to what is in Heaven. He was, however, having the Lord's outpouring love, peace, and comfort showering him with gold dust to protect him against Satan and any demonic entities while the surgeons were operating on him.

So, what exactly is gold dust? Some people reading this probably have no clue what this gold dust I speak of is. Here is the definition of "gold dust" that is classified as a Heavenly, spiritual, and supernatural phenomenon that comes from Heaven.

> *"Gold dust is a physical manifestation that arises from within the individual. Everything that's spiritual arises from within. The gold dust phenomenon, then, is a physical manifestation of a spiritual reality which is transmitted from a spiritual plane. Brethren, when someone has the Holy Ghost on them, and they pray healing for you and you're healed, that anointing arises from within the person that's praying, and it emanates from them. Healing virtue emanates from the person who*

Excerpt from Pastor Vitale's sermon from Living Epistles Ministries

My dad stated that it was such a phenomenal experience. It was so peaceful and so comforting. My dad told me that the gold dust he saw was the Holy Spirit speaking to him. It told him to turn around, at which time he saw a field in the distance. The Holy Spirit said the field represented his life. At which time, my dad put out his arms and said, "This is it!" To this day, we don't know exactly what my dad meant when he said, "This is it!" He doesn't even know, but he thought at the time he was crossing over into Heaven. He then saw my mom and I standing in front of him and cried out to the vision of my mom, "I don't want to leave you or Scotty!"

Upon waking up from surgery, my dad asked Pastor Mark about what the gold dust he saw was. Pastor Mark responded, "The streets of Heaven are made of gold." He thought his life was over. But it wasn't over. It is far from over. But then the next day, he wasn't alert. He wasn't awake or even his corny joking self. He was far from the same man that we were talking to the previous day.

On September 17, 2016, my mom and I went into my dad's hospital room to visit him. He wasn't himself. His left arm was trembling. It wasn't shaking all the time, but it was shaking randomly. My dad wasn't alert, but he'd move his right arm to stop it from shaking. It was a scary sight. He was alert in a minimal capacity, but barely able to speak where my mom knew that the trembling of his left arm was bothering him so she'd use her hands to try and stop it. I knew something was wrong from the start as he couldn't even move his left arm nor feel it. He couldn't even speak properly to tell us that he doesn't feel right. Besides, the left side of his face looked a tad slanted. I first thought of a simple acronym as the warning signs of something my dad may be suffering from: FAST. Fast stands for the following:

F: Facial drooping, a section of the face, usually only on one side, that is drooping and hard to move. This can be recognized by a crooked smile.

A: Arm weakness, the inability to raise one's arm fully.

S: Speech difficulties, an inability or difficulty to understand or produce speech.

T: Time, if any of the symptoms above are showing, then time is of the essence: call 911 or go to the nearest hospital.

I told the nurses what I have been noticing with my dad and they just shrugged it off as if he was just having an "off" day like Dr. Toms originally told us can happen. I wasn't buying it though! My dad had some good nurses, including Heather and Julie, who were the two nicest nurses of all and unfortunately, they both were off this day. I went up to his nurse and told her "Excuse me, but my dad isn't himself and I know the doctor said he'd have some good days and some bad, but his arm keeps shaking, he can barely speak, and his face is dropping on the one side. I also have observed that my dad cannot even move his left arm at all. As his son, I don't care what protocols there are to follow, something is not right with my dad and I want him to have an immediate MRI done to see if anything has gone wrong. If it comes back normal, then that is great. But if by chance something comes back abnormal, I want him to be checked so it can be fixed." The nurse, shocked at my stern tone of voice due to the love I have for my father, called for the doctor on duty to give him an MRI.

Thankfully, they gave him an MRI. The next day, the nurse on duty called my mom's cell phone as we were sitting in the cafeteria with a good family friend, Lynn. On the phone, she told us to hurry up to the Special Care Unit where they'll explain to us what has happened. My mom, Lynn, and I rushed to the SCU and the nurse on duty told us the MRI results came back. She told us that he suffered a major stroke and they are transferring him to the Intensive Care Unit (ICU) so he can be closely monitored, as when Dr. Toms comes in on Monday, they'll give him another MRI and then he may need to do surgery again to alleviate the swelling of my dad's brain. If he doesn't get the surgery, dependent on the secondary MRI come Monday, he could and most likely would pass away.

It was a long, long weekend for sure. I called the entire family and everyone came up to the hospital. Everyone slept over in the hospital's waiting room, which did turn into a fun time as the upcoming weeks progressed, which I'll explain why in a little bit. My cousin Sammi came up, as did my cousins Derek, and his girlfriend, Marissa, and Destinee. We even had visits from many family friends who came to see my dad, including Pastor Mike and Vikki. We had a lot of support for sure, but my dad just had a major stroke and we needed as much support, and more importantly prayers as we can get.

After everything that we went through and are continuing to deal with, such as this latest setback, my mom and I could barely eat or sleep. Besides, the waiting room we originally were in wasn't the most comfortable place to sleep neither. The chairs were so lightly-padded, but we found a more comfortable waiting room when my dad was transferred to ICU, and we made that our little nest, so to speak.

I have almost 5,000 friends on Facebook, which is the maximum number of friends you can have on the social networking site, and from one post about my dad's stroke, we had a grand total of 3,328 prayers (from the combined amount of likes/reactions and comments) and over 100 shares from various people worldwide.

My mom's friends were also praying for my dad after they found out about the stroke. As they were praying together on a Monday evening, like they generally do, they both received a message from the Lord that gave them the exact same and identical scripture from the Bible which says, "I shall not die, but live and declare the works of the Lord!" (Psalm 118:17) Let's put it this way, the power of prayer is most certainly a powerful thing and that is about to be shown and proven.

Since my dad had a stroke and not knowing what'll happen next. Not even knowing if my dad would live or die, I would get negative thoughts attacking my brain. I began conjuring all the "what if" scenarios that you could possibly think of, including "What if my dad dies?", "How would my mom and I go on with our lives without him?", and even "What if my dad never had the tumor discovered and we found him dead on the couch one morning?" All negative situations that never happened, but that Satan wanted to use to bring me down. Due to this, it led me into a downward spiral. I started going into a major depression, and it was becoming obvious that I wasn't myself anymore.

My aunt Candi told everyone, including my dad, that she was so proud of me for being so strong for my mom through this entire ordeal, so it was only fitting that Candi would be the one to help me kick out of my depression. She told me, "Your mom needs you now more than ever. You cannot let your mind and body shut down and claim defeat." She continued, "Your dad needs you too. He survived the surgery because you were so strong, so to survive this stroke, you need be equally as strong. If you stay depressed, your dad would feel like he was the reason your depressed and he will lose the power he has inside him to survive." I cried out to the Lord after talking to Candi and cast the depression put upon me by Satan and within minutes, my depression was gone and I was back to the strong man that I have been from the beginning. However, after I called out to the Lord to defeat the depression, my mom and I had an amazing surprise, yet my mom unaware until after I explained what I felt from the Lord's presence.

My mom and I were in the waiting room waiting for my dad to be transferred to ICU. The rest of my family was also present, but they all went together to go to the chapel to pray for my dad and that everything would come out alright. Something told my mom and I to wait for them to get back and not go along. This random guy enters the waiting room. He literally sits down right next to my mom and me. He is an older gentleman, and he was telling us this story of his son that was in a car accident. He began telling us of his Christian faith. He then asked my mom and I to join him in prayer after we told him everything my dad went through and is continuing to go through. Like seriously, what man in their right mind would ask two strangers, not knowing who they are, to pray in the type of society we currently are living in with people of Christian faith being prosecuted and murdered due to their beliefs.

After we prayed, we began talking some more about our personal lives. He was telling us of a dream he had, which I cannot remember as of this moment, however, I do remember the dream that he had was the exact identical dream that I had a few weeks ago. He then was telling us of his son and how he had certain characteristics that I won't get into due to them being identical to the characteristics I possess. Thing is, he'd have no clue that I possessed those same characteristics because he doesn't even know me, or does he?

I have no validity of what I suspect, even to this day, but having the same dream I had, the fact his son had the same traits I have, and that his son was in a car accident, I deeply and truly believe this guy was said son. I believe that he was this "son" that he said died in the car accident. In short, I believe that this guy was an angel who appeared himself to my mom and me. Not to mention, after looking at this guy from top to bottom, I have noticed cuts and lacerations on his knees which looks to have come from some type of accident which could have been put there as a way of God revealing this man as an angel to us.

After the rest of my family returned from the chapel, I asked my uncle Steve about this and he believes it to be true. He stated to me "Angels can take the appearance of human beings in the natural to give comfort and peace to other people that need such comforting and peace."

My dad got transferred to ICU and the entire family was in the waiting room, most of which slept over the entire weekend to await the results of the MRI first thing Monday morning, but I was terrified to leave his side. He wasn't alert yet and was technically in a coma due to the stroke to allow his brain to heal. Now, I've been in the hospital for roughly a week and a half straight without sleeping and not eating a thing. I know it wasn't the healthiest thing to do, but it's hard when you have someone you love going through so much and you are fearful of the "what if" scenarios.

My aunt Candi would take me home to go and freshen up. I remember vividly that when she was driving me home from the hospital to shower, a song would come on the radio. The song that came on was a sad song that would have me think of my dad and begin making me cry. I asked her to turn off the radio, and she did. She then brought me back to the hospital and I was back with the entire family as we waited for Monday to come to know what my dad's MRI shows.

When we first found out that my dad had a stroke on Saturday, I would call my entire family. I first called my uncle Steve who is close to the Lord. I mean, close is an understatement to be perfectly honest. He is a Christian counselor, as well as a prophet of the Lord. If you know my uncle, you would know that he is the most loyal son of our Lord and Savior, Jesus Christ. He is humble and would say that we all are loyal to our Lord, which is true, but my uncle lives on faith of the Lord in his everyday life and regarding his everyday decisions, especially the important and big ones. He has a strong relationship with the Lord, and after what I am about to tell you, you will too. The Lord is powerful, and if you don't believe that or are doubtful about that, then here is a testimony of something amazing that happened before we found out that my dad's stroke disappeared from the MRI results, something that even baffled Dr. Toms himself.

After I called Steve to tell him and my aunt Jeannette about the stroke my dad sustained, I called the rest of my family and everyone rushed down and slept over the hospital the entire weekend till we knew what'll happen and if another surgery would be necessary. On the way to the hospital, two days before my dad was going to get the secondary MRI, Jeanette heard God telling her to "Keep praising me!" She listened to the Lord and continued to praise him. As they continued driving to the hospital, my uncle Steve saw Jesus putting his hand in my dad's brain. He would go and pinch the brain bleed inside my dad's skull to stop the bleeding. He then released his fingers and the bleeding had stopped and the stroke and anything around it had been healed, including the cancer cells.

Two days later, Dr. Toms came in with his team and told us the results of the MRI and everything that followed. He said "He had a major stroke, a stroke that shows on the MRI that he shouldn't have survived. We thought we'd have to reopen his head to alleviate the brain's swelling so it doesn't explode within his skull." My mom, my uncle Steve, the entire family, and I look in astonishment, not sure what he's going to say next. Thinking my dad has either passed away or may need to have brain surgery, again, by alleviating the swelling of the brain. Dr. Toms continues "The most amazing thing has happened, something science cannot even explain, it was like it was a true miracle. Looking at the MRI, the swelling is gone. The brain isn't bleeding anymore. He did have a major stroke and will have temporary paralysis on the left side of his body, which he'll need to have physical, occupational, and speech therapies to heal and gain full mobility back, but it looks like the stroke has alleviated itself and some of the cancer cells that were lit up on the scan prior have been removed and killed from the stroke."

So, what do you know? Steve heard from the Lord that the bleeding had stopped two days prior to us getting the results back. A true miracle was witnessed by our entire family. Steve told us about what he saw Jesus do to the brain bleed two days prior to the MRI, and the results were synonymous with what Steve had told us. Dr. Toms even said from his own mouth that my dad's a true miracle as there were no scientific explanations on how the stroke and those surrounding cancer cells just miraculously disappeared like they did.

By the grace of God, my dad's stroke was miraculously healed over the course of a few days, and some simple prayers from amazing people worldwide, on top of the supernatural powers of our Lord and Savior, Jesus Christ, gave my dad his life. It just goes to show that the Lord doesn't want my dad in the Kingdom of Heaven just yet, which means that my dad has a purpose to yet fulfill on Earth and his time isn't up yet. He may have had some paralysis that would need to be given some rehabilitation, but the good news is that his life-threatening condition has become healed by yet another miracle from my Lord and Savior, Jesus Christ.

My dad was frustrated because he couldn't see too good. The tumor originally pushed away my dad's optical nerve in his brain, which is used to give him sight, and will take approximately a year or more to fully restore itself. He had no feeling on the entire left side of his body, which would eventually come back with some rehab at Geisinger HealthSouth's rehabilitation facility, as well as depression and emotional troubles. But who wouldn't be depressed, very sensitive, and even emotional after everything he has gone through and everything he will continue to go through for the next year. The memories of everything he has gone through, can be overcome by prayer, which, will be something he'll remember for the rest of his life.

My dad was staying in ICU for a few more days to be closely monitored to make sure that nothing will go wrong, again, and thankfully nothing did. In the waiting room, we must've had a party. The entire family slept in the hospital's waiting room for approximately two weeks or so straight, with some family members leaving late at night, and others spending the night on a rotating basis. We had tons of food in the waiting room. This waiting room was unlike those you would think of. There was a soda and snack vending machine, coffee machine, counters and sink, a kitchen table, comfy couches, a coffee table, a phone charging station for both iPhone and Android devices, etc.

Throughout our two weeks or so staying in this waiting room, my aunt Candi made her homemade macaroni and cheese with stewed tomatoes, my uncle Steve made his homemade soups, and we even ordered Domino's for delivery. We had approximately four or five bottles of two liter sodas, chips, pretzels, and snacks, and, of course, I had both of my laptops as I needed them to keep me occupied and my mind off what my dad was going through, not to mention I still had school to do, which, thankfully my professors were very lenient with me and extended my homework assignments. My assignments are usually due on Sunday nights, but my professors allowed my homework to be turned in by the last day of the semester with no penalties.

My dad asked the nurse a question all serious when he was being wheeled passed the waiting room we were "partying" in. He asked her "What is all that noise?" She responded "Oh, that's your family in the waiting room!" My dad replied, "It sounds like they are having a party." We were kind of having a party, a party for my dad's miraculous recovery and impending healing. My dad still tells this story to this day and says it with a smile on his face and laughing because he didn't want us to be sad and depressed the entire time he was in the state he was. The fact that both sides of the family, the McCoy's and the Seitzinger's, was something that made him happy. His brothers and sisters, his in-laws, his wife and son, and his nieces and nephews all fellowshipping and spending time together is something my dad was grateful for.

I remember one night, it was me, my mom, and my aunts Jeanette and Candi all sleeping in the waiting room one night. Jeanette and I love the two lifetime movies *Stalked by My Doctor*. There were two versions, the original being simply *Stalked by My Doctor* and then the sequel, *Stalked by My Doctor: The Return*. So, Jeanette and I watched it that night with Candi, who never saw it, and boy that was a fun night. We laughed during some scenes and just had a blast. I am so glad that our families got to spend time with each other. Our families always got along, we just never had time nor made time to get together, and ever since everything that has happened this past year, we have had roughly four or five picnics since the initial diagnosis. And I am sure there will be plenty more to come in the upcoming 2018 year.

My mom went to the restroom and my dad's nurse came into the waiting room where I was on my laptop doing some homework. While in the waiting room, I asked her if everything was okay, in a concerned tone of course, as it wasn't normal for a nurse to come to the waiting room to see the family if something isn't wrong. She told me, with a smirk on her face, and a chuckle in her voice, "Your dad wanted to buy your mom a dozen roses and have them delivered to the hospital and I was helping him, but his phone is dying so I was bringing it to the charger." I asked her why he wanted to buy my mom roses, and she responded "I asked the same thing, and he told me because she is my rock and has been by my side every step of the way. I know corny!" I laughed and said that's my dad for you!

I went to see my dad again, like I do approximately every five minutes to check up on him. He told me that the nurse said "You are so blessed to have a family that loves you. You have an entire waiting room of approximately 20 to 25 chairs filled with family." My dad responded "No, I'm the blessed one to have a family that cares so much." The thing is we are the blessed ones because my dad has done more than I can count for our entire family. It's just who my dad is. He thinks of others before himself, so to me it was no surprise that he had so many people that care for him. He's an amazing guy and the next year was all about us doing for him as he did for us all the years prior.

My dad was eventually transferred back down to SCU where he had Heather as his nurse again. My dad's roommate was another sign from God. He looked just like my pap and immediately approached my mom and me. We thought that it was a sign from God telling us that my pap is proud of how strong my dad is.

My dad kept asking us about the Bloomsburg Fair while in SCU. The fair ended about two weeks earlier, but due to everything his brain has sustained, he didn't even know it was over nor did we have the heart to tell him. He couldn't even tell time and didn't even know the month or date, because he needed to retrieve speech therapy from HealthSouth. The stroke did some major damage to his brain and he forgot even the simplest of things.

Every time my dad, mom, and I went to the Bloomsburg Fair, we'd always get the famous hot sausage hoagies from there. Well, after everything my dad's brain has been through, his brain still remembered those hot sausage hoagies! HA! He kept asking for someone to bring him back a hot sausage hoagie from the fair or if we can take him. We said he cannot go, but we will bring him one back. We wouldn't bring him one back, and eventually, after a few days, he'd drop the subject. We just didn't want to tell him the fair was over and break his heart. It may sound small, but after everything his brain has been through, he was and currently is to this day very sensitive and emotional.

A day or so later I would go back in to check on my dad in one of my every five minute visits. I walked in on something frightening. My dad had two nurses, Heather and Julie, in his room and he kept shaking. I wasn't sure what was happening, whether it was a seizure, his heart was stopping, or something. I wasn't entirely sure, Heather tried calming me down with her words, as she and Julie helped him get warm. Thankfully, it was nothing major, he just had a urinary tract infection (UTI) because of the catheter they used on him due to him being classified as a "fall risk." Those few minutes though were scary for me to see my dad shaking and not knowing what was happening with him. It was just something so unexpected, but thankfully it wasn't anything major and wasn't another setback. That's all we'd need is another setback, but thankfully that wasn't the case.

My dad continued to show his concern for others, despite himself. Because of how the nurses took such good care of him, he wanted to repay them for their gratitude. It was their job, but he doesn't care if they were being paid to take care of him, he sees them as a human being who sincerely showed care to him as their patient. He was about to be discharged from SCU and moved to a normal room for a few days, where they'd not monitor him as often. He was so worried to be removed from SCU, because he wanted to get the nurses there Centiole's Pizza. Time after time, he kept asking when the pizza was coming to make sure they got their reward for taking good care of him. Thing is, Centiole's Pizza, which closed for a few years and was reopening, wasn't opened for business yet and unfortunately, we were unable to get the nurses the pizza my dad wanted to get for them. He was a tad disappointed, but just like they say, "It's the thought that counts!"

After my dad was moved down to a normal room, he was later discharged after being cleared of all life-threatening conditions and setbacks. Where does he go from here? It is time to go to Geisinger HealthSouth's rehabilitation facility where his road to recovery begins...

CHAPTER 4: ROAD TO REHABILITATION

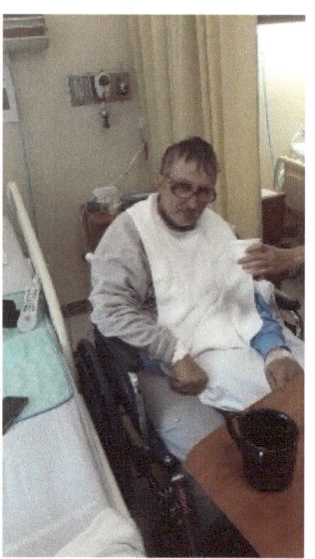

My dad was transferred to Geisinger HealthSouth's rehabilitation facility where he would begin his road to rehabilitation. Here he'd obtain intense physical, occupational, and speech therapies.

We were no longer in the actual Geisinger hospital, so my uncle Dave and aunt Marci were kind enough to lend us their drivable RV. We spoke with Geisinger's security officers and they agreed to let us park right up the hill from HealthSouth so my mom and I could sleep comfortably and relatively close to my dad, who was staying inside a hospital room in the rehabilitation facility where he'd remain monitored. The security guards gave us a "police escort" of sorts to show us exactly where we could park the RV and made sure the rest of the security guards were made aware of them giving us permission to park the RV on Geisinger property.

I would stay over a few nights, but mostly my mom slept in the RV with one other family member who'd spend the night on a rotating basis. I thought since my dad was doing better with no more setbacks to happen, I would be okay going back home and finally letting everything that had happened so quickly set in and have my time alone to grieve, cry, and talk to the Lord just to understand the past few weeks of hardships my family had been going through.

I would visit my dad usually two sometimes three times a week with hitching a ride off my aunt Lou Ann, since she literally lives right down the street from me. Upon hitching a ride, I'd spend the entire day at the rehabilitation facility with my dad before being taken back home by Lou Ann.

It was hard seeing my dad vulnerable and unable to do things he was always capable of doing, primarily walking. My dad would be in a wheelchair where he was wheeled around by the nurses, at least until he would relearn how to walk and do physical exercises during physical therapy. He even had to go to doctor appointments at the main hospital unit down the road. HealthSouth had a van for my dad to take that would transport him to and from the main hospital where he had his appointments. When his appointments were almost done, my mom would call the van's number and they'd pick them up and transfer them back to the rehabilitation facility.

One thing my dad despised about the place was the fact that he had to take salt pills. The salt pills were necessary for him to take as it would decrease the swelling in his brain. Without them, the swelling wouldn't go down which would make the rehabilitation process not completely work as he'd not obtain the proper mobility at the pace needed.

The nurse asked my dad if he likes applesauce, to which he stated he does. She then asked if he liked potato chips and he responded back that he does. She told my dad to pretend it is applesauce flavored potato chips. She told him this, because they crush up the salt pills and put it in his applesauce. This was necessary, since he was still undergoing speech therapy and wasn't fully capable of swallowing pills yet. My dad took the salt pills by eating the applesauce and he responded back to the nurse "Lady, that didn't help!" When my dad told us that story, we all laughed. Oh, and to this day, my dad cannot eat applesauce and he used to love it!

My uncle Joe was always visiting my dad. He'd not miss a day of the week to come and visit my dad. He'd be right by my dad's bedside from morning until early afternoon. Joe went through a difficult time the past couple of weeks as he watched my dad fight for his life. The past few years, Joe's life was quite difficult and heartbreaking. He lost his parents, his brother, Ken, and his best friend and wife, Mary Ann. He didn't want to see something else happen to another family member, and he was by my dad's bedside the entire time as much as possible for hours a day, even watching college football games with him.

It was also a nice surprise for my dad when my great-uncle Roni, who is my mom's uncle, came to see my dad. Roni hitched a ride off Lou Ann and Kirk which really cheered up my dad because they are super close to each other.

My dad, in HealthSouth, was very stubborn. He just wanted to go home and get out of the hospital, but was in no condition to do so. My uncle Kirk told him from his experience in the hospital "Scott, I did whatever the nurses told me to do. I ate what they told me to eat. I drank what they told me to drink, and I listened to everything they said because if I did, I'd get better and go home." That sunk into my dad's brain as he kept repeating it to us daily. Within time, he was sent home, but not until his grueling rehabilitation program to become stronger both physically and mentally was completed.

The first couple of days there my dad wanted to go to the bathroom. He's the type of person that does what he wants when he wants and doesn't want help from those around him as he is extremely independent. He tried to get out of his bed and the nurses heard him and they came to stop him as he cannot even stand on his own yet. He fell and knocked down approximately six nurses to the ground as they tried to stop him from falling and injuring himself even more. That plan backfired, however, as the rest of his stay at HealthSouth consisted of him having an alarm put underneath him, whether it be in his wheelchair or in his bed. It did backfire, but ultimately my dad became stronger from physical and occupational therapy.

My dad had to learn everything over again while at HealthSouth. He had to learn how to tell time again, count numbers, walk, eat, go to the bathroom, sit up, get dressed, and even remember dates and the days of the week. He had to relearn the simple things that you take for granted in everyday life and don't think much of doing, but it takes a lot for your brain to comprehend. I never knew it took so much for the brain to comprehend these types of things, but when you suffer from a brain tumor, and then have a stroke afterwards, your brain goes through so much turmoil, wear, and tear. It technically is being reprogrammed, and it is like you are starting life over again, as if you were toddler in an adult's body. My dad even said to us many times that he feels like a child in a man's body.

Pastor Mike and Vikki came to visit my dad at HealthSouth. They asked my dad, "What do you want us to pray for, Scott?" My dad responded, "I cannot open my left hand, can you please pray for that?" So, we all laid hands on my dad and prayed along with Pastor Mike that my dad could open his left hand. Unlike before, he immediately began to open his left hand, which just goes to show that praying is a powerful thing as Christ answered our prayers.

He sometimes got frustrated with the rehabilitation process, and would try to take the easy way out or do things on his own. I caught him doing this a few times, and in return, I was called a snitch for the time I told his occupational therapist that he was cheating during his memory exercises. I only did so because I didn't want him to have to go through this awful ordeal again, and secondly, I wanted him to get better and cheating would just prolong the success rate of his rehabilitation.

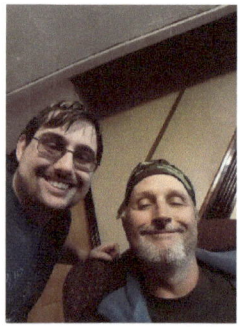 Exactly one month after surgery, which took place on September 15, 2016, he was released from HealthSouth. It was October 15, 2016 and my dad has come home. He had some restrictions and had to be watched like a hawk because he isn't the type of person to just sit around and do nothing. He hated having others wait on him hand and foot. He is an extremely independent person, but he had no choice. He took care of us so many times, now it was our turn to take care of him. However, he was still getting outpatient rehabilitation and beginning his next adventure: beating cancer itself.

CHAPTER 5: KICKING CANCER'S ASS

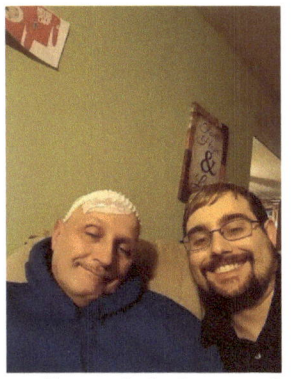 Upon being released from HealthSouth and coming home on October 15, 2016, we had to install some specialty items in the home, such as a bar by the toilet, a bar in the shower, and put some mats in the shower so my dad wouldn't slip with the water hitting the shower's floor. Ultimately and thankfully, it was some minor adjustments, but well worth it for my dad who has come a long way, yet has a long way to go.

Even though he was released from HealthSouth and Geisinger as a patient, he still had to do some outpatient therapy for physical and occupational rehabilitation, as well as outpatient radiology to remove and kill any remaining cancer cells that were in his brain, which was approximately 1 to 5 percent. While at home, he'd have to do some memory games and brain teasers for his brain to reprogram itself, as well as lift small weights, do some squats, and even do some other physical activities to regain full mobility back on the left side of his body.

I can be a tad overprotective, especially since he was free from the nurses and he thought he can do anything he wanted unsupervised. But boy was he wrong! It's funny though, as my dad was still his funny, sarcastic self. While I watched him like a hawk, my dad came up with a few other nicknames for me on his road to recovery.

As I stated earlier, I earned the nickname, "snitch" for ratting him out to his occupational therapist. Well, while he got released from the hospital, I earned a few new nicknames. I was called a drill sergeant for forcing him to continue his exercises at home on his off days from his physical and occupational therapies at HealthSouth. I also got called a policeman because I wouldn't let him get off the couch without telling my mom; which he claimed made him feel like he was under house arrest. I remember my dad getting off the couch to do something, as he's not the kind of guy to just lay around and do nothing, and I yelled to my mom, "Mom, he moved!" My dad looked at me and sarcastically said to me, "You little squealer!"

I only did all this because I care about my dad and I didn't want him to fall or get hurt. I knew he would try to do something he couldn't do on his own, but would normally do if he wasn't in this type of situation. However, I may have been a tad too strict on him from time to time, but only for his own well-being. Some may call it "tough love" and that's all it was, just so he wouldn't get himself into trouble.

My dad got frustrated when he got released from the hospital and couldn't do the things that he originally could do. When tax season came around, we even had to hire an accountant, because his memory wasn't good enough to deal with the numbers. He didn't like hiring an accountant, because he always did the taxes himself, and this year was no different. After all, he is the man that wants to provide for his family. There were plenty of miniscule things that my dad wanted to do but he couldn't. That irked my dad, because he felt it was his job to provide for his family and not have my mom or someone else do it for him.

While doing outpatient radiation and rehabilitation, my parents would stay at a place owned by Geisinger called the House of Care. The House of Care is a place for cancer patients that can stay for a low fee. It is cheaper than a hotel room, but only for Geisinger patients that have been diagnosed with some form of cancer. It is like the Ronald McDonald house, and they'd shuttle my mom and dad to his appointments and treatments.

My aunt Lou Ann and uncle Kirk were so nice and supportive during this whole crazy journey we have been on, as were the rest of our family, and still are to this very day. They were so kind that they even paid for the first week of my parents stay at the House of Care. That meant so much to me and my parents. It means more to us than they would even know and we were and still are extremely grateful for their loving and generous gesture.

My dad would enjoy getting up early in the morning and watch Newswatch 16, which is our local news station. My mom would not let my dad go off on his own, so he wandered off one time without my mom's knowledge and ended up getting lost. My dad, confused due to everything his brain has gone through, couldn't remember where the room he was staying in was at. He'd sit on the step for two hours waiting for someone to come to him so he could ask where to go. No one would come out, so he had to guess which room was his and thankfully, the room he chose was the correct right. After telling me this story, he said "It was such a lucky guess!"

When my dad began his radiation treatments, I told him that there was only one thing I wanted this year for Christmas. Christmas was a month or so away and I just wanted my dad to be cancer free. I didn't need any gifts, money, or anything, just my dad to no longer have any cancer. That's all I ever wanted to get for Christmas, but would I receive that gift?

Let's put it this way, my dad had an MRI halfway through his radiation treatments, usually around the third week of radiation or so. We received the results the day before Thanksgiving. These results stated that my dad needed to finish the remaining treatments of radiation, however, all his cancer cells have been obliterated completely and he was 100 percent officially cancer free. The scientific word calls it "remission," we as Christians call it a "healing."

On Thanksgiving 2016, we shared the news with the entire family. The only ones who new prior to Thanksgiving were my uncle Steve, aunt Jeanette, my mom, my dad, and I. But on Thanksgiving 2016, we shared this amazing news with my nana, great-uncle Roni, aunts Lou Ann and Lesley, uncles Kirk and Ron, and my cousins Derek and Sammi. I would then call my aunts Marci and Candi, and my uncle Joe and let them know the amazing news. Afterwards, I would let the world know the amazing news we just received by posting a status on Facebook.

Thanksgiving is classified as a holiday to give thanks and be thankful for all that you have. I didn't just get my early Christmas gift, but a gift to be thankful for. Thankful for my dad's recovery, survival, and now becoming cancer free. It's only fitting to receive amazing news on Thanksgiving. A holiday to give thanks, and we gave thanks to the Lord. This Thanksgiving we had A LOT to be thankful for and without the Lord's help and strength, none of this would have been possible.

My dad has a stubborn side to him, as do all the McCoy's. My dad is tenacious and stubborn and he used that tenacity and stubbornness to not let cancer win. To beat cancer. To kick cancer's ass, if you will. Cancer has met its match in Scott George McCoy. Satan tried everything he had. His most powerful curse was that brain tumor and then the stroke that followed, but Satan's most powerful curses were no match for the Lord's love and strength that he instilled within my father. My dad may be strong, but it is thanks to our Lord and Savior, Jesus Christ, that my dad has become cancer free. Satan's inability to keep my dad down just proves how much more powerful the Lord is and Satan was made to look like an evil fool.

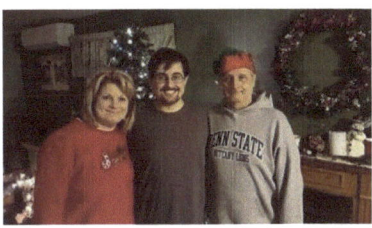

On Christmas Eve, my mom's side of the family always gets together to celebrate, fellowship, and exchange gifts. I didn't care what gifts I got as I already got my gift, my dad becoming cancer free and being able to join us on Christmas Eve this year. When this all happened, we didn't know if my dad would live or die. We had faith he'd survive, but anything was possible. Thankfully through the miracles of Christ, my dad did what we knew he could do and that being the obliteration of cancer and more importantly, the defeat and ultimate humiliation he put on Satan. He showed Satan that he could do all evil to our family, but Christ will always prevail victorious in the end and we won't allow ourselves to be tortured, tormented, defeated, and manipulated by something as wicked and evil as him. And as we prayed, "Through Jesus stripes, my dad is healed!" And that he was, he was healed!

The coming months, we had our ups and downs as a family. My dad started the Optune device, which sends electromagnetic waves into my dad's brain. Whenever the cancer cells divide, it would create and regrow the tumor. However, with the Optune device, it'll kill any dividing cancer cells and zap them with the electromagnetic waves, killing them, thus not allowing the tumor to regrow.

Unfortunately, one major setback was the fact that my uncle Joe, who was my dad's brother, fell and broke his artificial hip. He had to undergo hip replacement surgery, and due to complications from the surgery, he had passed away on March 13, 2017.

Just a few days before Joe passed, my aunt Marci was visiting him in the hospital and she told me that he said, "Scott went through so much, too much." As he said this, he turned his head and wiped a tear from his eye. Marci told me she saw her grandfather, my great-grandfather's, face in him.

Due to Joe's passing, my dad was depressed. Joe did so much for my dad, including transporting him and my mom to his treatments. My dad was grateful for the time he got to spend with Joe, both in the hospital and on the commutes to and from his appointments. But my uncle is in a better place and I'm sure he is singing the praises of the Lord with his wife, my aunt Mary Ann, as well as his parents, my grandparents, and his brother, my uncle Ken. I am sure they are rejoicing with the Lord for looking over my dad during this entire ordeal he had gone through and helping him defeat Satan. And I am sure they will continue to praise the Lord in Heaven, as the Lord continues to look over my dad, and bless our family for many years to come.

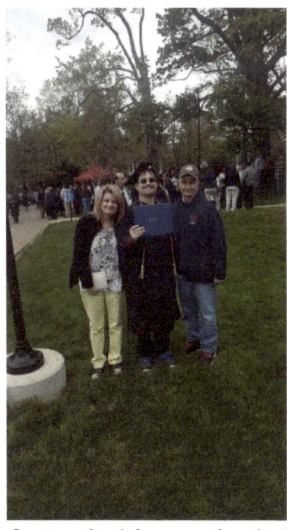

As I stated previously, I contemplated dropping out of college. My dad said the best medicine was for me to graduate so he can attend my commencement ceremony. In May 2017, my dad made it to my commencement ceremony in Burlington, Vermont. I graduated from Champlain College with a Bachelor's of Science Degree in Web/Software Development. My dad's determination to see me obtain my degree I worked so hard for was a factor in his survival, fight, and speedy recovery.

I am proud to state as of September 14, 2017, exactly one year after my dad was diagnosed with Glioblastoma, my dad is still cancer free. My dad's most recent MRI, the one year MRI, was on September 21, 2017 and he received the results the same day and the results came back as negative. This means the cells are still stable and no cancer cells began to regrow or divide. My dad will have to get an MRI every two months for the rest of his life, unfortunately. However, as of November 2017, it marks one year that my dad was announced cancer free. Dr. Turner, who was taking over for Dr. Toms, told my dad that he has plenty of years left on his life with the way things are currently progressing.

My dad has beaten all the odds that the doctors feared he wouldn't be able to overcome in his lifetime, including things such as driving and cooking. My dad drives. He even drove two hours to my apartment and he did amazingly well! My dad cooks. To be honest, my dad loves to cook and I hate to say this, but his cooking before all this happened was awful. Well, not really, he was an amazing cook, but after this all happened, I must say his cooking somehow seems to have gotten even better. He has made some of his best dishes after his surgery, which makes my dad happy to hear. My dad agreed with me after one batch of BBQ he made. It was simply phenomenal. I'm glad to finally hear that my dad is beginning to see what I do.

We still reminisce and laugh at how we took over the lobby and waiting rooms. It was quite fun, despite the horrible situation we found ourselves in. Sometimes I felt we were enjoying ourselves too much when we were "taking over" the waiting rooms at the main hospital unit. The reason for this was the bonding of our families (both my mom and dad's side of the family).

The revelations of everything that was going wrong were starting to take a turn for the best and good things began happening. Due to this, and of the miracle we saw, helped us relax, laugh, eat, sleep, talk, watch movies, and yes even cry at random times together as a family. Close family friends even stopped by with food and drinks for us, which made us realize we don't have just a good and close family, but we also have an amazing set of friends.

My mom and I are always emotional when it comes to bad and tragic events that happens to those close to us. We only got through this awful ordeal with the love, hope strength, and peace the Lord has given us. Even though Satan tried to attack our family, we knew that God was much more powerful and due to this belief and faith we had, which was strengthened throughout the past year, our faith and belief in the Lord Jesus led to Satan's ultimate defeat and humiliation.

Through all these setbacks, came some obstacles to overcome. Through all this darkness, came some light. Through all this evil that Satan tried to throw at us, came some purity through the Lord, Jesus Christ. As it states in the Bible, "I can do all things through Christ which strengthens me." (Philippians 4:13)

My dad is a hero. He is a Christian and a man of God. If you just have belief and faith in the Lord, you can then be shown the light and the way. It just goes to show that miracles do happen. My dad is living proof of that! I saw it with my own eyes and heard it with my own ears that my dad is a miracle from Dr. Toms himself.

This book is a direct testimonial from myself to prove to everyone that if you don't have Jesus Christ as your Lord and Savior, it isn't too late to do so. Just ask him into your life. My dad's life was on the line, and I put all my faith into Jesus. I was terrified, scared, and fearful, all signs of the enemy. But Jesus helped me get through that and because of my faith being strengthened as it was, I became a stronger Christian and my dad defeated cancer; yet more importantly *Christ Defeated Cancer*.

PICTURES

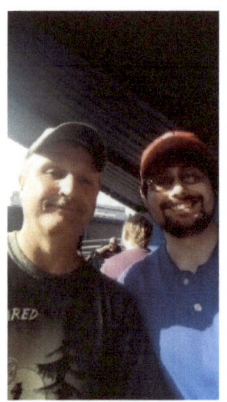
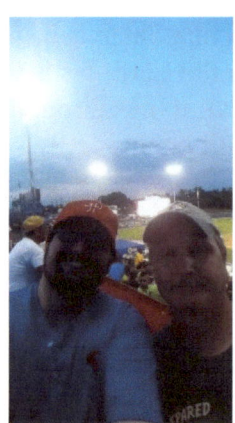
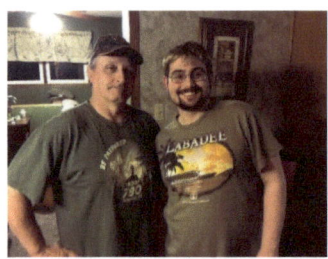
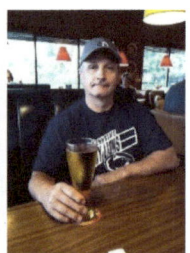
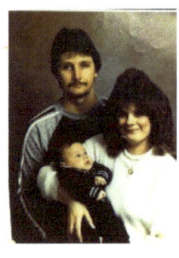
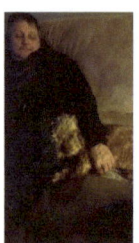
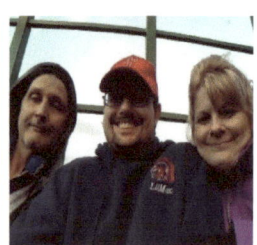

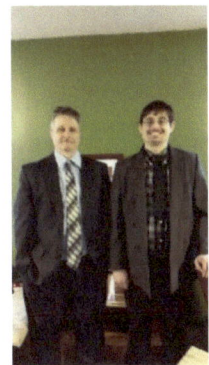
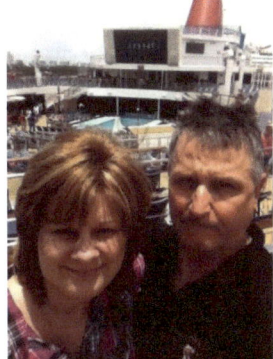
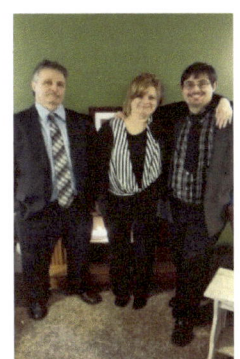

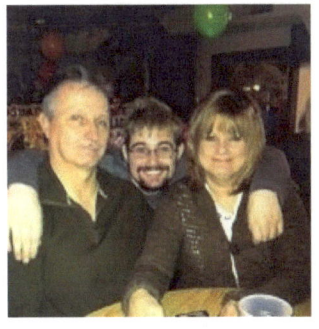
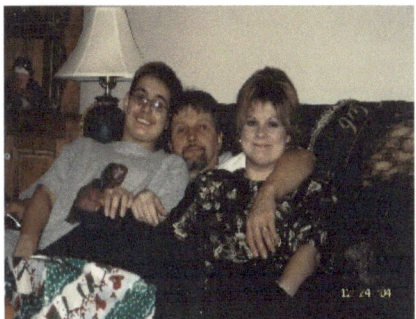

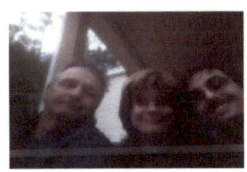
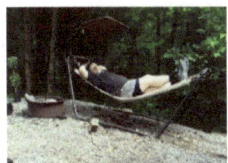
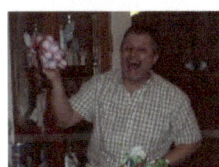

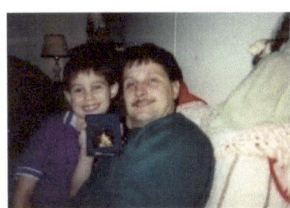
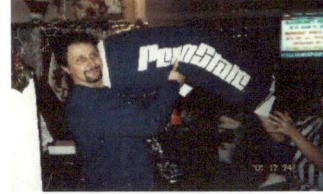
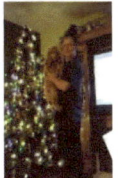

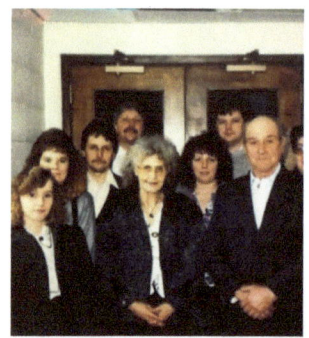
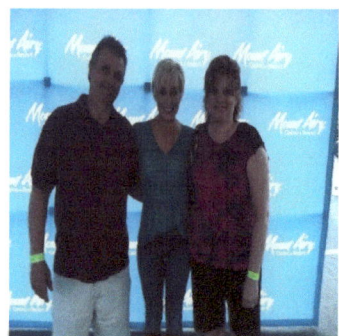

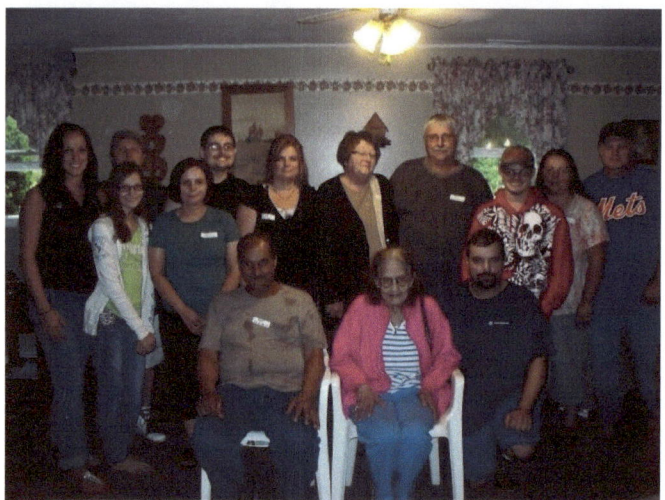

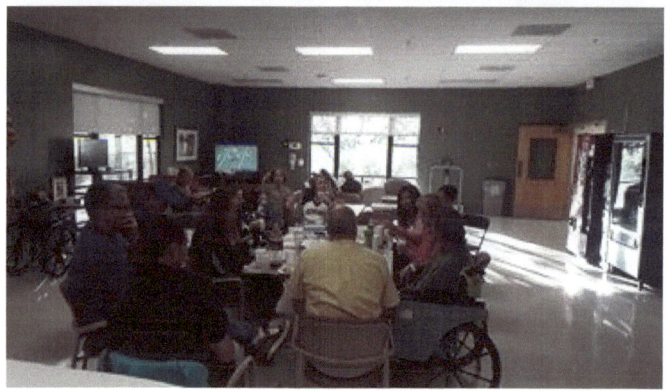

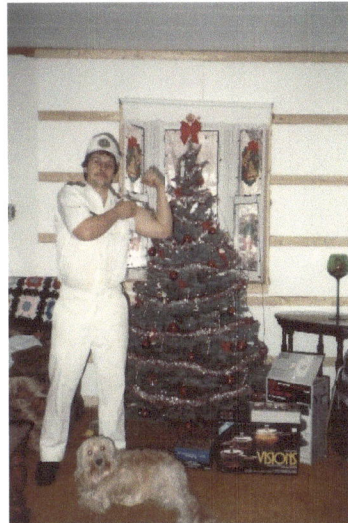
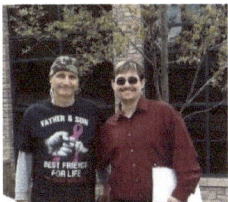
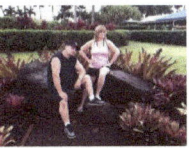
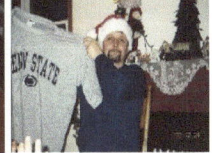
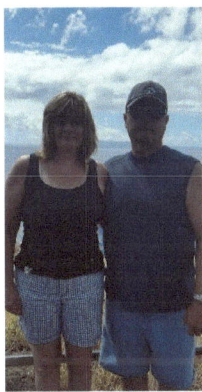
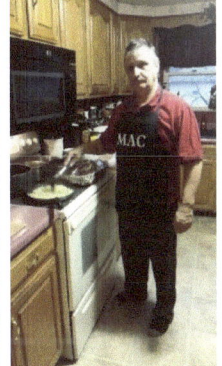
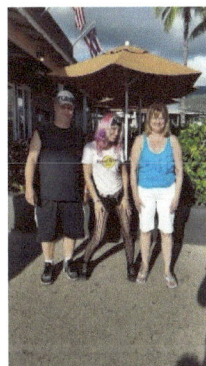

"Christ Defeats Cancer"   Scotty McCoy

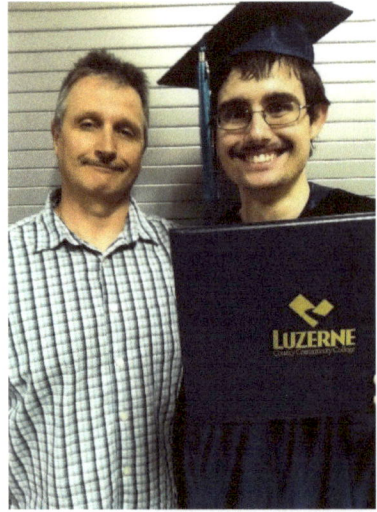
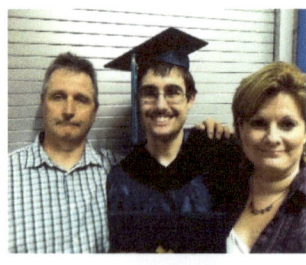
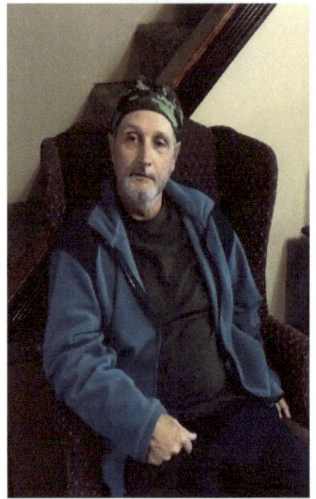
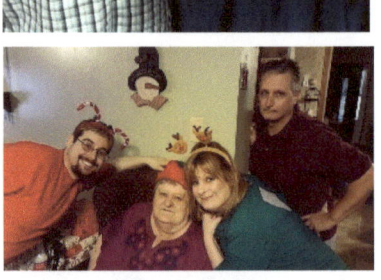
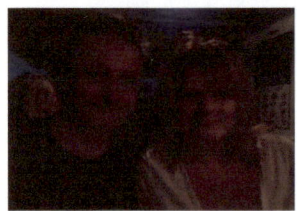
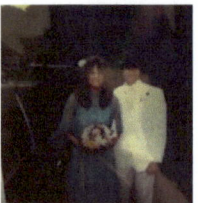
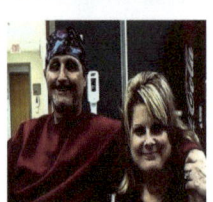
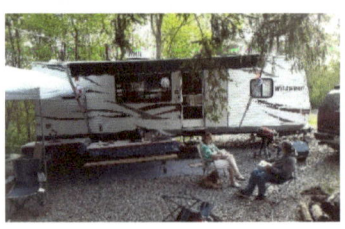
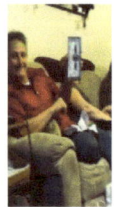
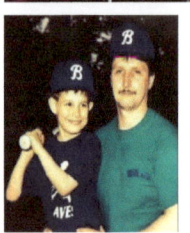

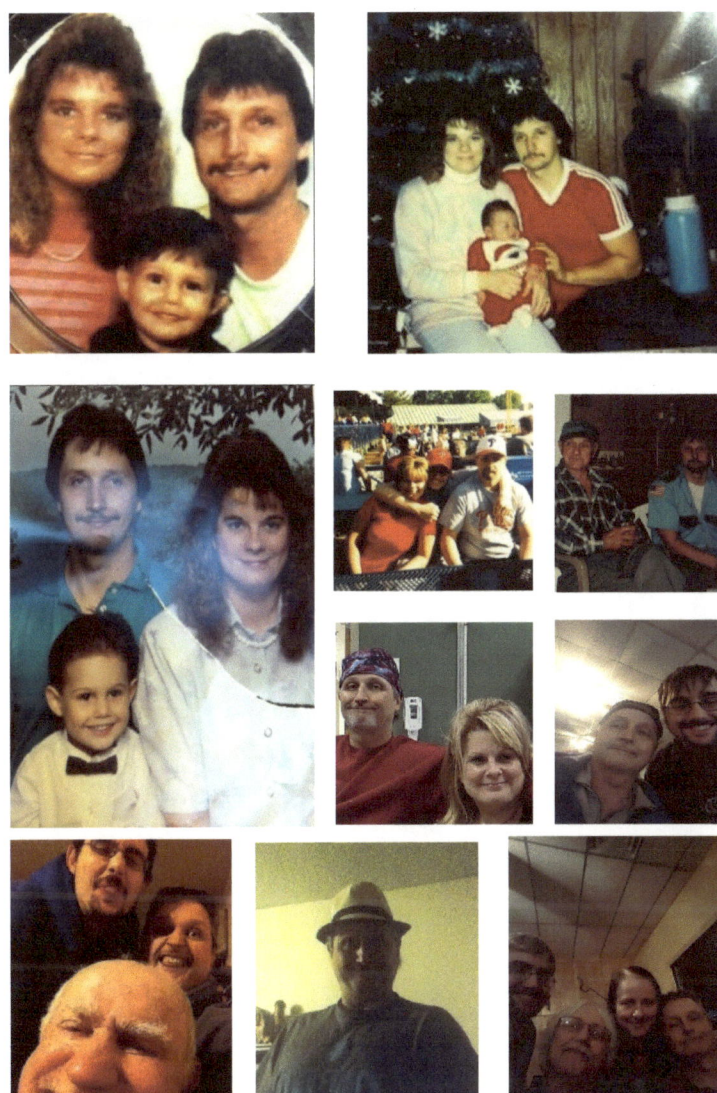

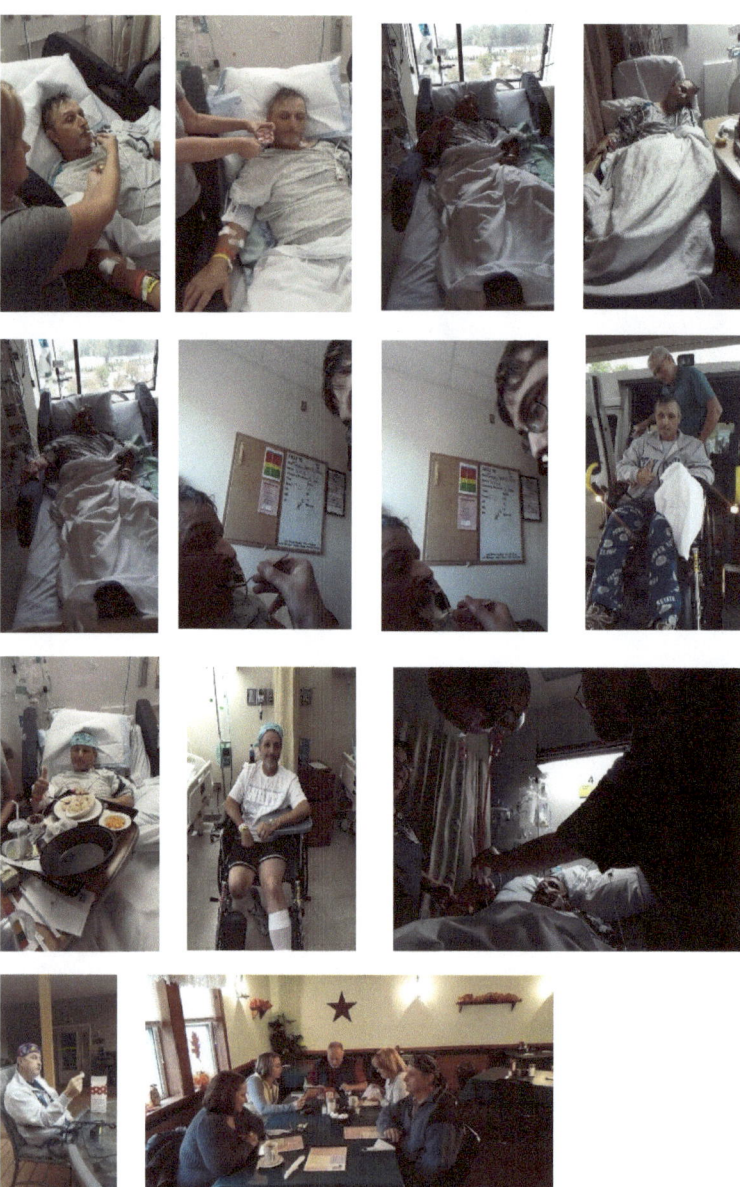

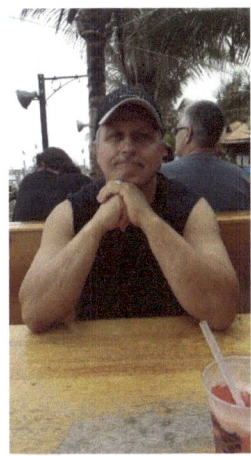
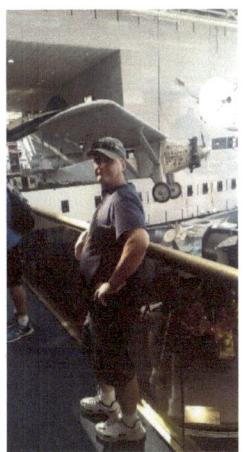
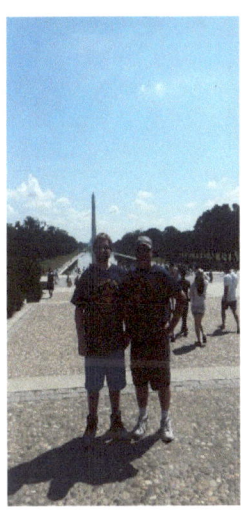
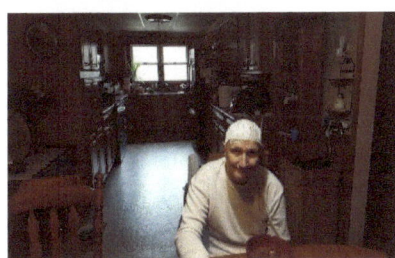
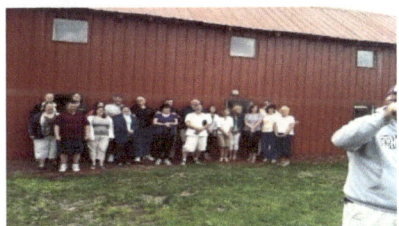

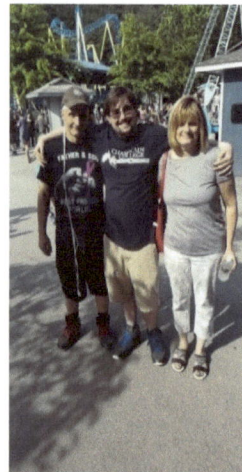
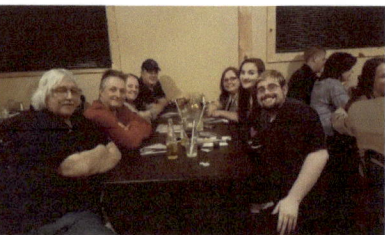
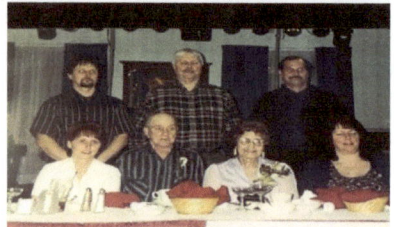
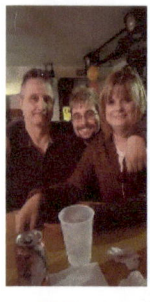
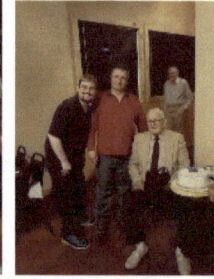
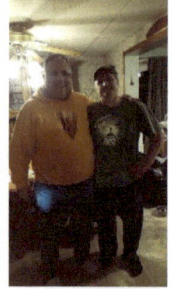
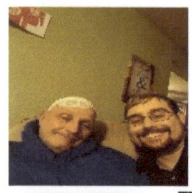
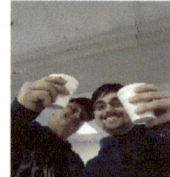
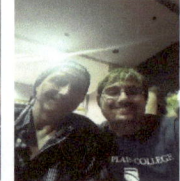
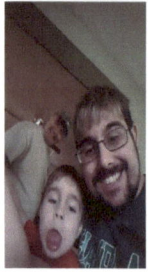
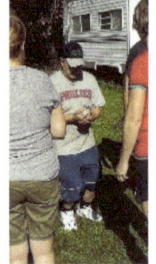
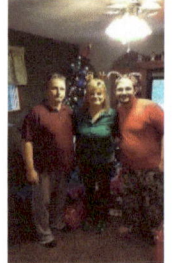

MCCOY MEMORIAL

Rest in peace to all my dad's side of the family that have crossed over into the Kingdom of Heaven to be with our Lord and Savior Jesus Christ.

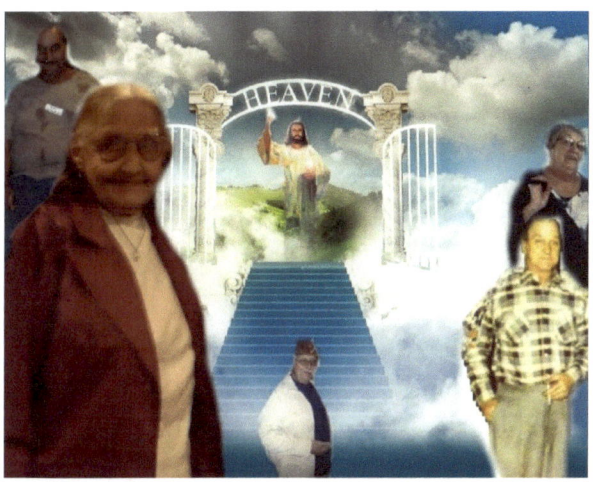

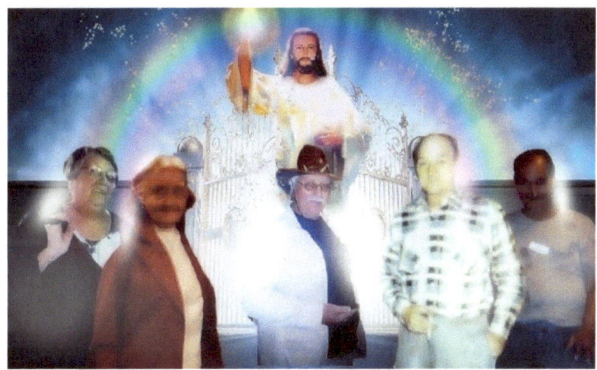

CONTACT

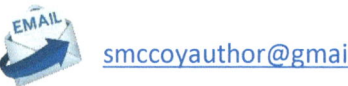 smccoyauthor@gmail.com

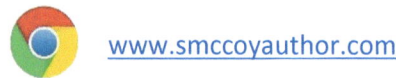 www.smccoyauthor.com

SOCIAL MEDIA LOUNGE

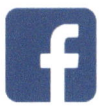 www.facebook.com/smccoyauthor

 www.twitter.com/smccoyauthor

 www.instagram.com/smccoyauthor

www.ingramcontent.com/pod-product-compliance
Lightning Source LLC
Chambersburg PA
CBHW040320010626
45792CB00024B/2077